# SPANLINGO

# SPANISH FOR PHARMACISTS

## Georgia Patilis

**IN LOVING MEMORY OF MY FATHER,**

**ANDREW PATILIS**

Dear Dad,

This book is dedicated to you, with my deepest love and respect for the selfless sacrifices that you made for your family. You worked countless hours to make sure that your children would have the education and opportunities that were not availed to you.

Andrew Patilis, my dad, my hero. Not like the ones in the movies. A real life hero, who sacrificed his own dreams so that his children would have a better life. Your love for your family knew no bounds. Your family was your core and you led by love and example.

May you Rest in Peace in Heaven.

# INDEX

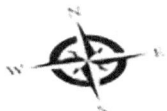

# DIRECTIONS TO THE PHARMACY-DIRECCIONES A LA FARMACIA

North→norte

South→sur

East→este

West→oeste

## Traffic Signs→ Señales de tráfico

| Turn to the left. Doble a la izquierda. → Turn to the right. → Doble a la derecha. | Go straight ahead. → Vaya derecho. | Yield. →Ceda el paso. | Cross the street. →Cruce la calle. | Turn right/ left at the traffic light. → Gire a la derecha/ a la izquierda en el semáforo. |
|---|---|---|---|---|
| Stop sign → el signo de alto / señal de stop | One Way→Una vía | No Parking. →Prohibido estacionarse | Speed Limit→Límite de velocidad | U-Turn→ Hacer una vuelta en U |

## KEY DIRECTION WORDS

Avenue→ *la avenida*

Block→ *la cuadra*

Corner→ *la esquina*

Intersection→ cruce

Roundabout→ *la glorieta, el redondel*

Sidewalk→ *la banqueta*

Sign→ *el rótulo*

Street→ la calle

Traffic light→ el semáforo

## DIRECTION VERBS

- **INSTRUCTIONS TO PATIENT**

| | |
|---|---|
| Cross → Cruzar | Cruce… |
| Go towards→ Ir hacia | Vaya hacia… |
| Go through→ Atravesar | Atraviese… |
| Go past→ Pasar al lado | Pase al lado… |
| Turn →Doblar | Doble… |
| Turn around → Dar la vuelta | Dé la vuelta… |
| Turn off the highway→Salirse de la autopista | Sálgase de la autopista… |

# PATIENT PRELIMINARY INFORMATION- INFORMACION DEL PACIENTE

## PHARMACY CARD →TARJETA DE FARMACIA

Do you have a pharmacy card? → ¿Tiene tarjeta de farmacia?

Can I see your pharmacy card? → ¿Me puede mostrar su tarjeta de farmacia?

Do you have a pharmacy savings card?→ ¿Tiene una tarjeta de ahorros / tarjeta de descuento en farmacia?

Do you have a Rx Savings plan? ¿Tiene un plan de ahorros Rx?

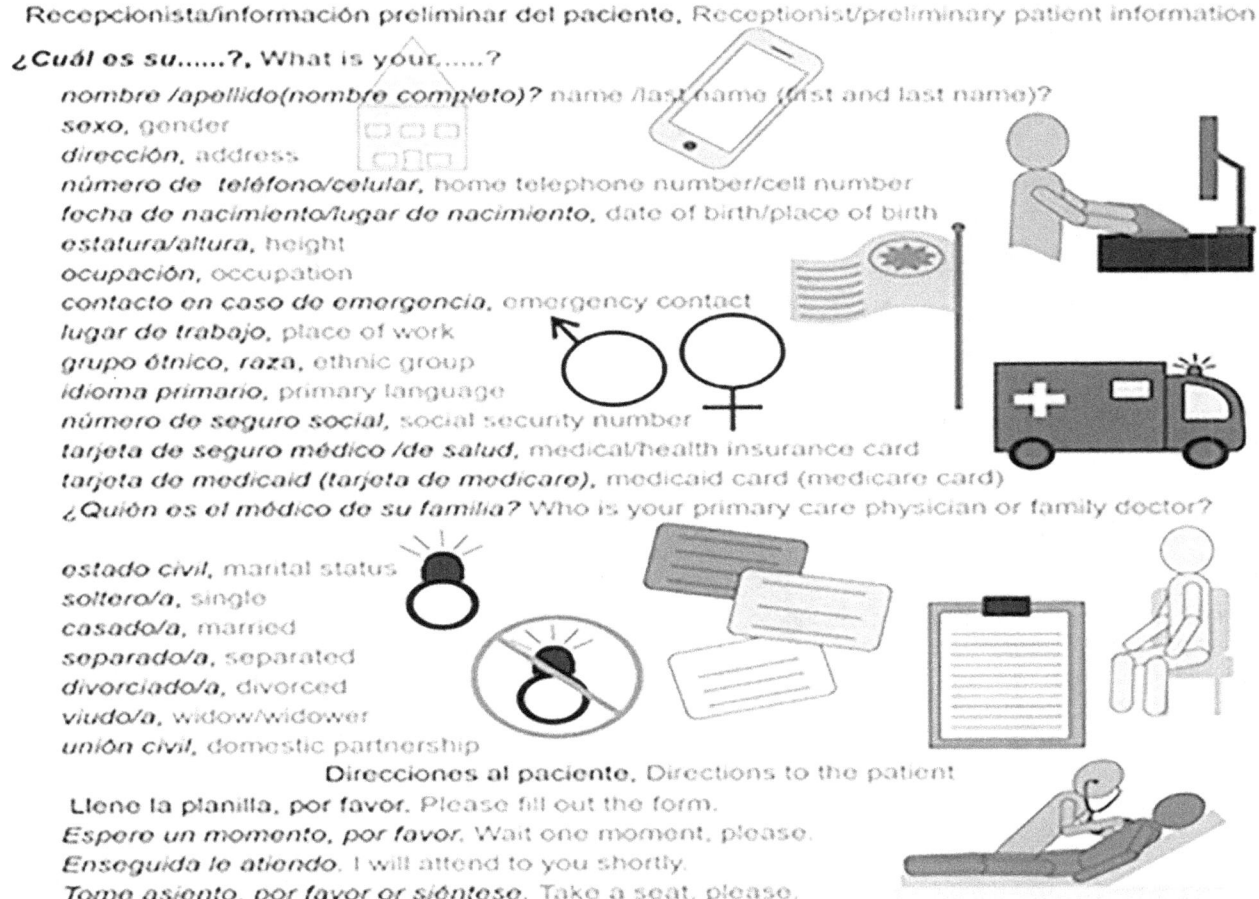

Recepcionista/información preliminar del paciente. Receptionist/preliminary patient information

*¿Cuál es su......?,* What is your......?

*nombre /apellido(nombre completo)?* name /last name (first and last name)?
*sexo,* gender
*dirección,* address
*número de teléfono/celular,* home telephone number/cell number
*fecha de nacimiento/lugar de nacimiento,* date of birth/place of birth
*estatura/altura,* height
*ocupación,* occupation
*contacto en caso de emergencia,* emergency contact
*lugar de trabajo,* place of work
*grupo étnico, raza,* ethnic group
*idioma primario,* primary language
*número de seguro social,* social security number
*tarjeta de seguro médico /de salud,* medical/health insurance card
*tarjeta de medicaid (tarjeta de medicare),* medicaid card (medicare card)
*¿Quién es el médico de su familia?* Who is your primary care physician or family doctor?

*estado civil,* marital status
*soltero/a,* single
*casado/a,* married
*separado/a,* separated
*divorciado/a,* divorced
*viudo/a,* widow/widower
*unión civil,* domestic partnership

Direcciones al paciente. Directions to the patient

Llene la planilla, por favor. Please fill out the form.
*Espero un momento, por favor.* Wait one moment, please.
*Enseguida le atiendo.* I will attend to you shortly.
*Tome asiento, por favor or siéntese.* Take a seat, please.

# PATIENT MEDICAL HISTORY

Present medical history (illnesses), Historia médica enfermedades

Do you drink alcohol? ¿Usted bebe alcohol?
Do you use recreational drugs? ¿Ingiere drogas recreativas?
Do you smoke? ¿Usted fuma?
What are your hobbies? ¿Cuáles son sus pasatiempos?

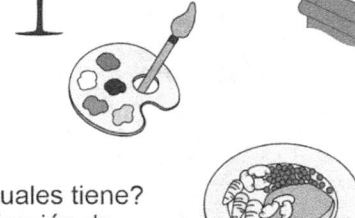

Are you pregnant? ¿Está embarazada?
Have you ever been pregnant?, ¿Ha estado embarazada?
Are you sexually active? ¿Está activo(a) sexualmente?
How many sexual partners do you have? ¿Cuántas parejas sexuales tiene?
Do you have a sexually transmitted infection? ¿Tiene alguna infección de transmisión sexual?

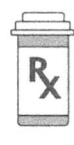

Do you have allergies...? ¿Tiene alergías...?
to any food/any medicine/any antibiotic? a algún alimento/a alguna medicina/algún antibiótico?

Have you ever had any of the following illnesses? ¿Ha tenido alguna de las siguientes enfermedades?

Has any member of your family had any of the following illnesses?¿Algún miembro de su familia ha tenido alguna de estas enfermedades?

Is there anyone in your family with … ? ¿Hay alguien en su familia con … ?

·Alzheimer's disease, La enfermedad Alzheimer
·blood clots,coágulos de sangre
·cancer, cáncer
·type of cancer, tipo de cáncer
·diabetes mellitus/diabetes type 1/diabetes type 2, diabetes mellitus/ la diabetes tipo 1/la diabetes tipo 2
·epileptic attacks, ataques epilépticos
·heart attack, ataque de corazón
·heart disease, enfermedad cardiovascular
·heart problems, problemas del corazón
·high blood pressure, presión sanguinea alta/la presión arterial alta

·high cholesterol, colesterol alto
·migraines, migrañas
·Multiple Sclerosis, Esclerosis Múltiple
·paralysis, parálisis cerebral
·stroke, derrame cerebral or infarto

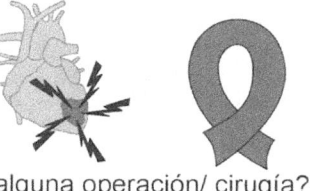

Have you had any surgery? ¿Ha tenido alguna operación/ cirugía?
Other hospitalizations? ¿Alguna hospitalización?
Other serious illnesses? ¿Alguna enfermedad grave?
Other serious injuries? ¿Alguna herida grave?

Vaccine Information, Información sobre sus vacunas

Do you have all your vaccinations completed?/Do you have all your vaccines? *¿Tiene sus vacunas completas? ¿Tiene todas sus vacunas?*

Have you received the vaccine for... ¿Recibió la vacuna contra...?
...Hepatitis A ? Hepatitis B? ...la hepatitis A? ...la hepatitis B?
...pneumococcal?...la neumocócica?
...chickenpox? ...la varicela?
...MMR? (Measles, Mumps, Rubella), contra MMR? ...triple vírica? (el sarampión, las paperas y la rubéola)
...shingles? ...la culebrilla?
...smallpox? ...la viruela?
...rabies? ...la rabia?
...COVID 19? ....Covid 19?

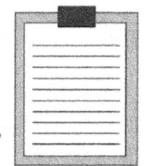

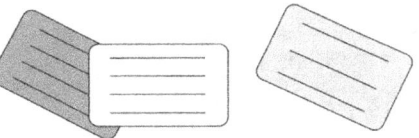

Which one are you missing? Which ones are you missing? ¿Cuál le falta? ¿Cuales le falta?

Do you have your vaccinations records (card)? ¿Tiene su registro (cartilla) de vacunación?

OJO *take note* : The World-wide Day of Celebration for Pharmacists-El Día Mundial del Farmacéutico is celebrated on September 25th. This was established by the Federación Internacional Farmacéutica o *FIP.*

# RX-PRESCRIPTION LABEL

Instructions for medication, Instrucciones para medicamentos

Prescription Label, La etiqueta

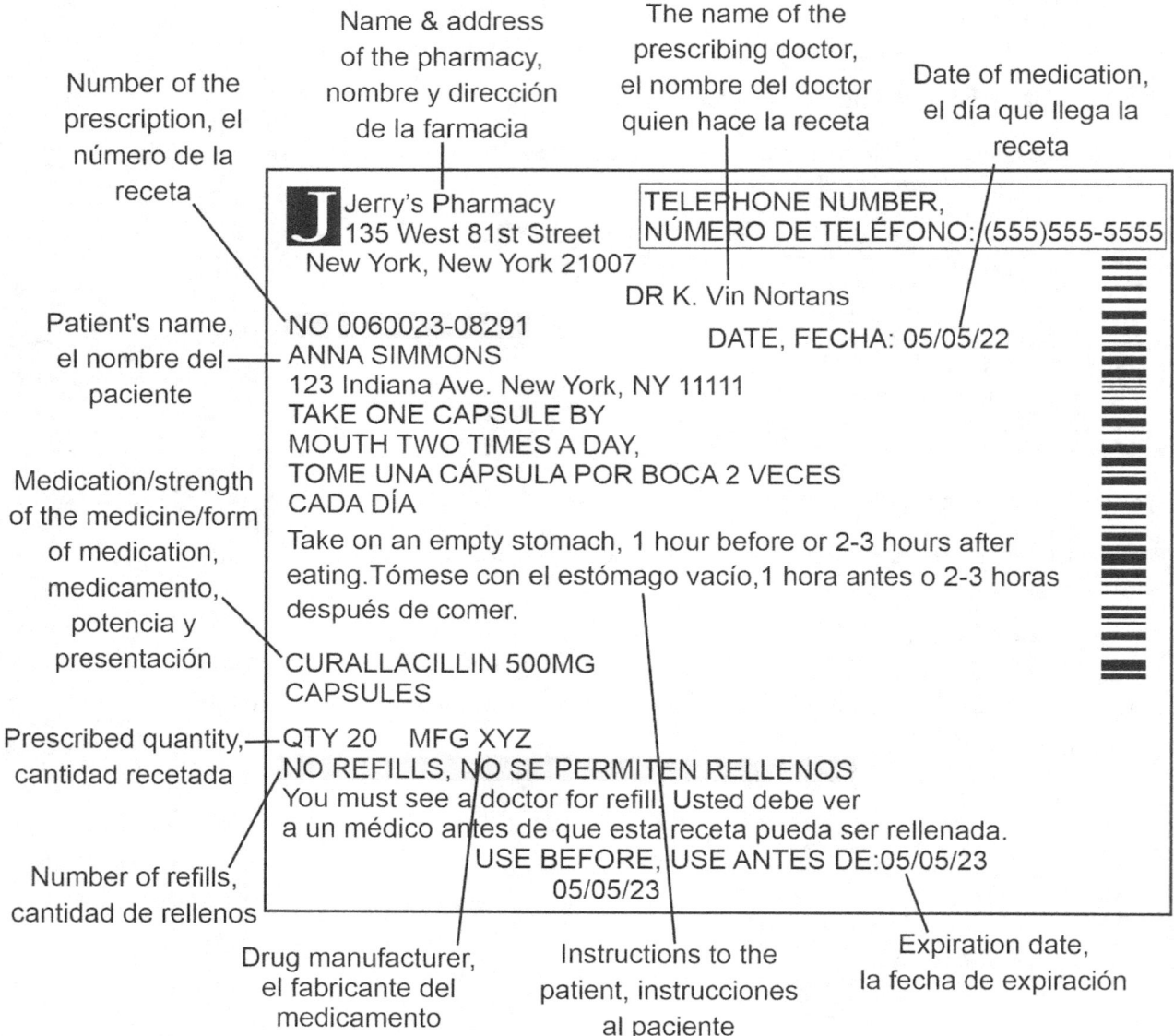

Number of the prescription, el número de la receta

Name & address of the pharmacy, nombre y dirección de la farmacia

The name of the prescribing doctor, el nombre del doctor quien hace la receta

Date of medication, el día que llega la receta

Patient's name, el nombre del paciente

Medication/strength of the medicine/form of medication, medicamento, potencia y presentación

Prescribed quantity, cantidad recetada

Number of refills, cantidad de rellenos

Jerry's Pharmacy
135 West 81st Street
New York, New York 21007

TELEPHONE NUMBER, NÚMERO DE TELÉFONO: (555)555-5555

DR K. Vin Nortans

DATE, FECHA: 05/05/22

NO 0060023-08291
ANNA SIMMONS
123 Indiana Ave. New York, NY 11111
TAKE ONE CAPSULE BY
MOUTH TWO TIMES A DAY,
TOME UNA CÁPSULA POR BOCA 2 VECES
CADA DÍA

Take on an empty stomach, 1 hour before or 2-3 hours after eating. Tómese con el estómago vacío, 1 hora antes o 2-3 horas después de comer.

CURALLACILLIN 500MG
CAPSULES

QTY 20    MFG XYZ
NO REFILLS, NO SE PERMITEN RELLENOS
You must see a doctor for refill. Usted debe ver
a un médico antes de que esta receta pueda ser rellenada.
USE BEFORE, USE ANTES DE: 05/05/23
05/05/23

Drug manufacturer, el fabricante del medicamento

Instructions to the patient, instrucciones al paciente

Expiration date, la fecha de expiración

OJO take note : A study (**Accuracy of Computer-Generated, Spanish-Language Medicine Labels** by Iman Sharif, MD, MPH; Julia Tse, BA, *Pediatrics* (2010) 125 (5): 960–965.) evaluated the accuracy of computer-generated translation of medicine labels in Spanish. The research was conducted in pharmacies around Bronx, New York and involved 316 independent pharmacies. Researchers evaluated 76 medicine labels generated by 13 different computer programs commonly used by pharmacies. The study found an overall error rate of 50 percent.

- One example of a prescription mistranslation was that of a man with a heart condition whose prescription stated that his medication should be taken **once a day**. The English term **once** is read as "once" (on-se), which is the Spanish word for the number 11. As the English instruction was retained in the medicine label, the **patient mistakenly took 11 pills** rather than just one pill per day.
- Misspelling in the translations created hazardous and potentially life-threatening errors. For example, the word "poca", which means "little", instead of the word " boca", which means "mouth". Another example of a misspelled error is "dos besos", which means "two kisses", instead of "dos veces", which means "two times".
- Poor translations specifically cited in the study included: "Take 1.2 aldia give dropperfuls with juice eleven to day.""Taking 0.6 mL 2 times to the day by the little with juice." "Apply to affected area twice to the indicated day like."

# MEDICATIONS

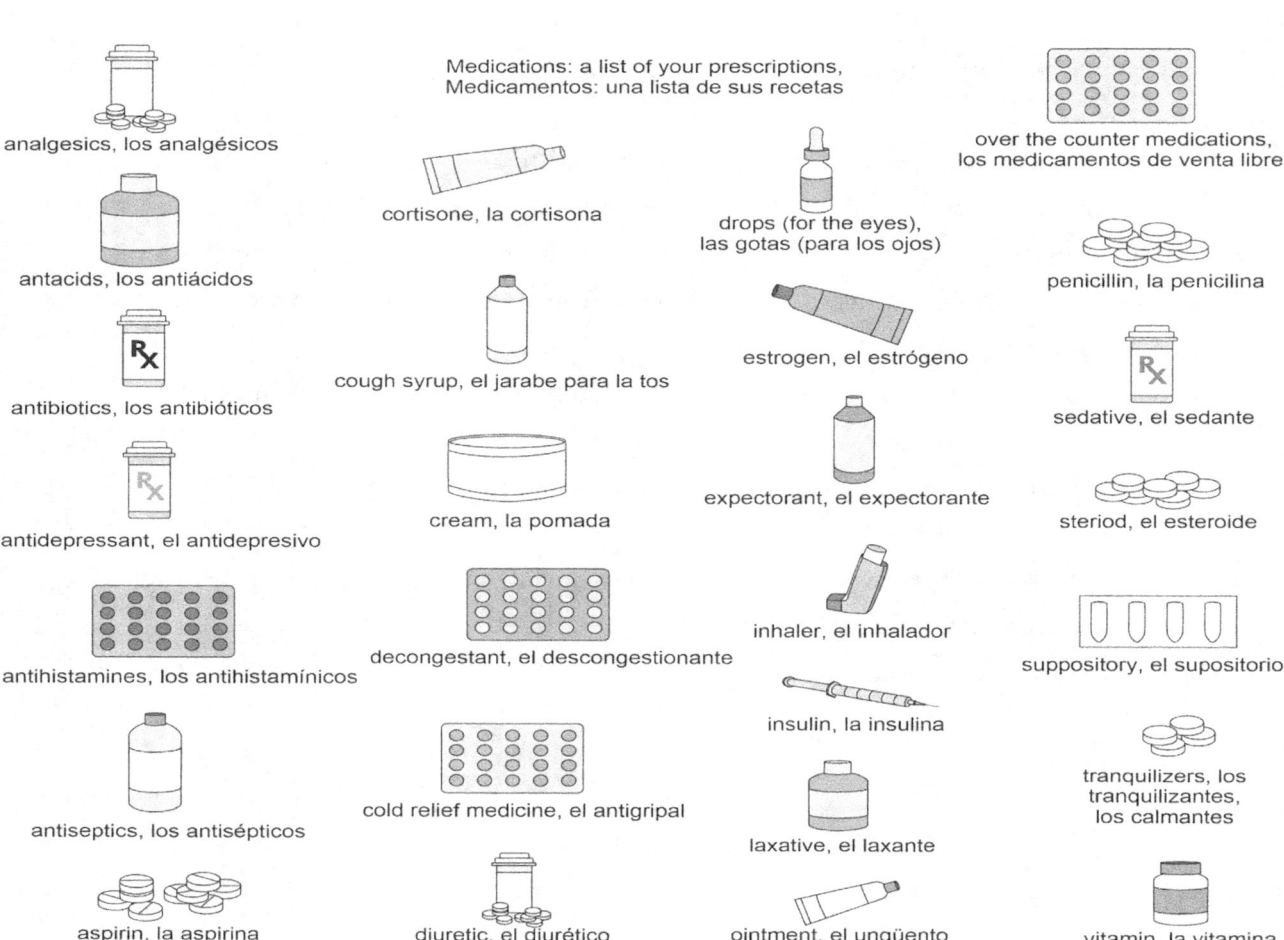

analgesics, los analgésicos

antacids, los antiácidos

antibiotics, los antibióticos

antidepressant, el antidepresivo

antihistamines, los antihistamínicos

antiseptics, los antisépticos

aspirin, la aspirina

Medications: a list of your prescriptions,
Medicamentos: una lista de sus recetas

cortisone, la cortisona

cough syrup, el jarabe para la tos

cream, la pomada

decongestant, el descongestionante

cold relief medicine, el antigripal

diuretic, el diurético

drops (for the eyes),
las gotas (para los ojos)

estrogen, el estrógeno

expectorant, el expectorante

inhaler, el inhalador

insulin, la insulina

laxative, el laxante

ointment, el ungüento

over the counter medications,
los medicamentos de venta libre

penicillin, la penicilina

sedative, el sedante

steriod, el esteroide

suppository, el supositorio

tranquilizers, los
tranquilizantes,
los calmantes

vitamin, la vitamina

## UNITS OF MEASURE

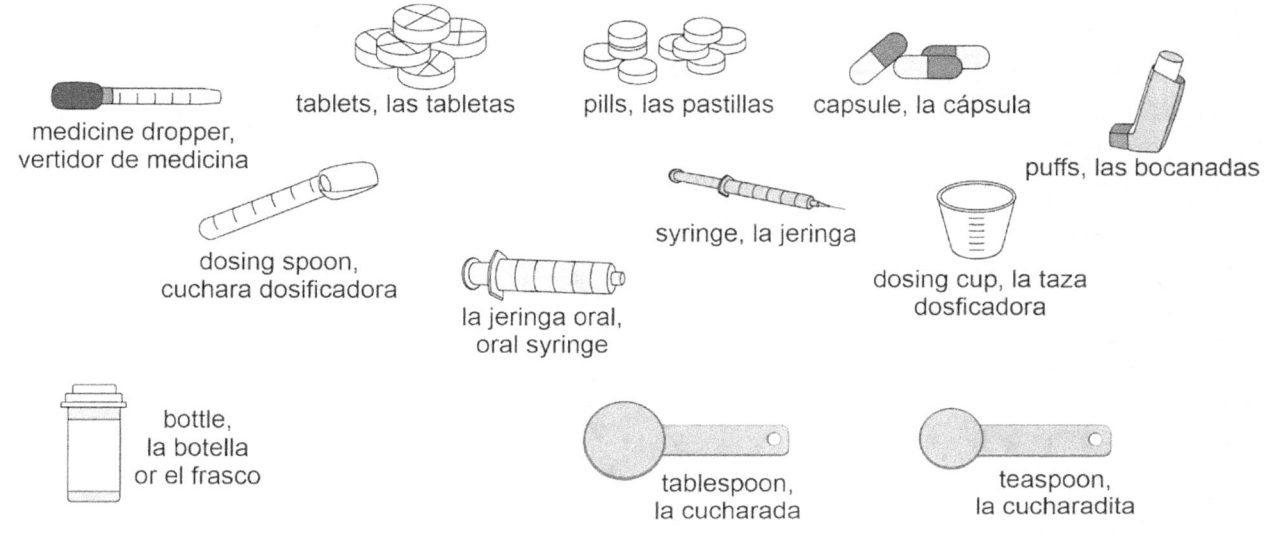

Units of measure, Unidades de medida

medicine dropper,
vertidor de medicina

tablets, las tabletas

pills, las pastillas

capsule, la cápsula

puffs, las bocanadas

dosing spoon,
cuchara dosificadora

syringe, la jeringa

dosing cup, la taza
dosficadora

la jeringa oral,
oral syringe

bottle,
la botella
or el frasco

tablespoon,
la cucharada

teaspoon,
la cucharadita

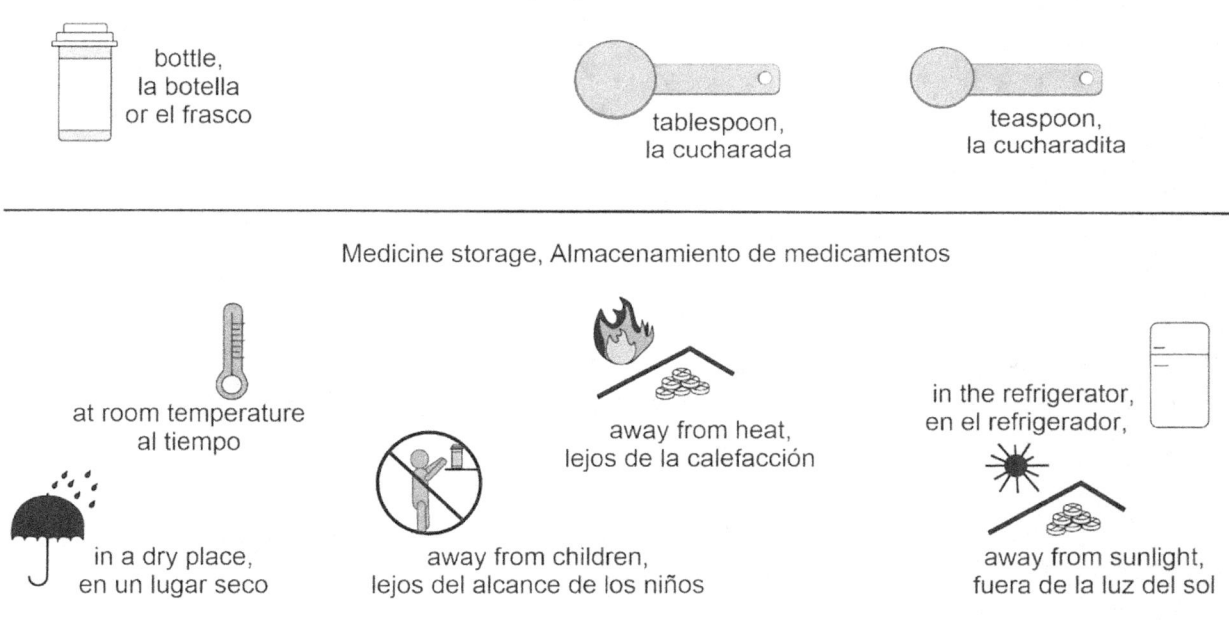

Medicine storage, Almacenamiento de medicamentos

at room temperature
al tiempo

away from heat,
lejos de la calefacción

in the refrigerator,
en el refrigerador,

in a dry place,
en un lugar seco

away from children,
lejos del alcance de los niños

away from sunlight,
fuera de la luz del sol

# METHOD OF INGESTION

Method of ingestion, Como ingerir
To swallow, tragar
To chew, masticar
To put drops in eyes, poner gotas
To inhale, inhalar
Inhaler, el inhalador
Injectable, el inyectable
Nasal use, uso nasal
Nasal inhalers, inhaladores nasales
Oral inhalers, inhaladores orales
Oral use, uso oral
Pump, bomba/bombilla

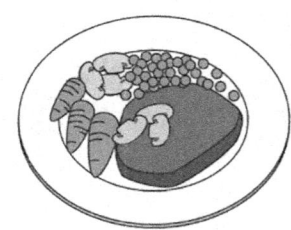

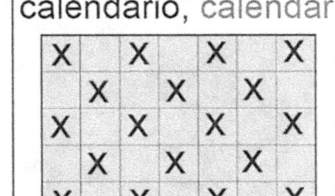

calendario, calendar

Frequency, Frecuencia
Take this medicine…, Tome estamedicina
____times a day, ____veces al día
Every day…every other day….., cada día ….un día sí, un día no, cada tercer día
Every___hours, cada ___ horas
in the morning/evening, por la mañana/por la noche.
Before eating /with each meal/after eating…, antes de comer/con cada comida/
después de comer

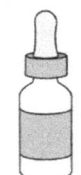

How to Take Medication, Instrucciones para tomar la medicación
On an empty stomach, en ayunas/ Tómeselo con el estómago vacío
With plenty of water, con mucho agua
Don't chew; swallow, No lo mastique
Don't take with alcohol. No tome con alcohol.
Don't drink milk or dairy products while taking this medication. No tome leche o
productos lácteos mientras esté tomando esta medicina

## Warnings, Advertencias

Avoid staying in the sun while taking this medicine. Evite exponerse al sol mientras esté tomando la medicina

Chew pills before swallowing.  Masticar antes de tragar.

Keep in a cool place. Consérvese en un lugar fresco y seco

Keep out of reach of children.  Manténga los medicamentos fuera del alcance de los niños

Keep refrigerated. Manténgase refrigerado/a.

Shake well before using.  Agítese bien antes de usarlo.

You need to take all of the medicine. Necesita tomar toda la medicina.

## Side effects, Efectos secundarios

This medicine can cause…, Este medicamento puede causar

diarrhea, diarrhea

dizziness, mareos

drowsiness, somnolencia

dry mouth, boca seca

stomach pain, dolor estomacal

This medicine can impair driving, Este medicamento  puede afectar la capacidad para conducir

## Refills/Expiration, Rellenos/Fecha de caducidad

Expired medication, medicamentos caducos

Expiration date, Fecha de caducidad/fecha de vencimiento

This medicine does not have refills. Esta receta no puede rellenarse.

Throw out after _____, Deséchese después  de………

There can be _____ refills. Esta receta puede _____ rellenados

Don't use after _____, No use después de_____

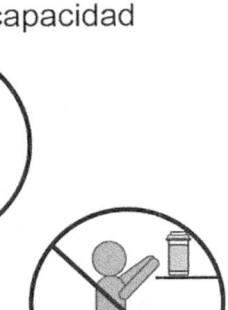

# SAMPLE RX LABELS

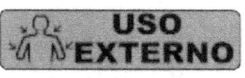
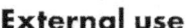

**USO EXTERNO**

External use

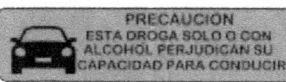

TÓMESE CON BASTANTE **AGUA**

Take with enough water

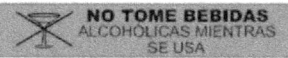

NO TOME BEBIDAS ALCOHÓLICAS MIENTRAS SE USA

Don't drink alcoholic beverages while taking this

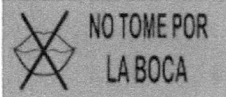

NO TOME POR LA BOCA

Don't take by mouth

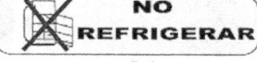

PRECAUCIÓN ESTA DROGA SOLO O CON ALCOHOL PERJUDICAN SU CAPACIDAD PARA CONDUCIR

Warning: This drug alone or with alcohol can harm your hability to drive

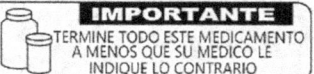

TOME ESTA MEDICINA CON EL ESTÓMAGO VACIO 1 HORA ANTES O 2 Ó 3 HORAS DESPUES DE COMER

Take this medicine on an empty stomach, 1 hour before, or 2 or 3, hours after eating

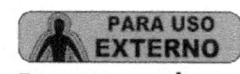

NO USE DESPUES DE FECHA: _____

Don't use after Date: _____

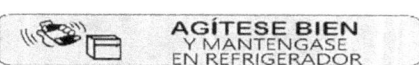

MANTENGASE FUERA DEL ALCANCE DE LOS NIÑOS

Keep out of reach of children

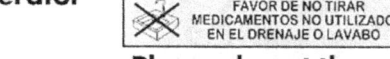

NO REFRIGERAR

Do not refrigerate

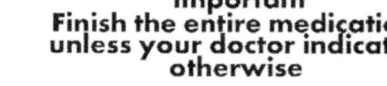

**IMPORTANTE** TERMINE TODO ESTE MEDICAMENTO A MENOS QUE SU MEDICO LE INDIQUE LO CONTRARIO

Important Finish the entire medication unless your doctor indicates otherwise

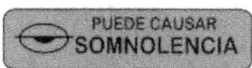

PARA USO EXTERNO

For external use

AGÍTESE BIEN Y MANTENGASE EN REFRIGERADOR

Shake well and keep in refrigerator

FAVOR DE NO TIRAR MEDICAMENTOS NO UTILIZADOS EN EL DRENAJE O LAVABO

Please do not throw out medications not used in the drain or sink

PUEDE CAUSAR SOMNOLENCIA

Can cause drowsiness

NO TOME CON JUGO TOME CON AGUA O LECHE

Do not take with water or milk

ESTE **Rx** PUEDE RELLENARSE 1 2 3 4 5 6 7 8 9 10 COMO SEA NECESARIO

Can be refilled as needed

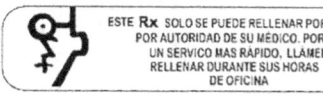

ESTE **Rx** SOLO SE PUEDE RELLENAR POR POR AUTORIDAD DE SU MÉDICO. POR UN SERVICO MAS RÁPIDO, LLAMENOS RELLENAR DURANTE SUS HORAS DE OFICINA

This RX can only be refilled by your doctor for faster service, call in your refill during office hours

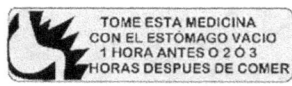
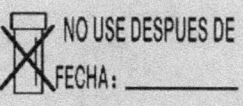

OJO *take note* : There is a green cross outside of pharmacies in Spain.

# FIRST AID KIT

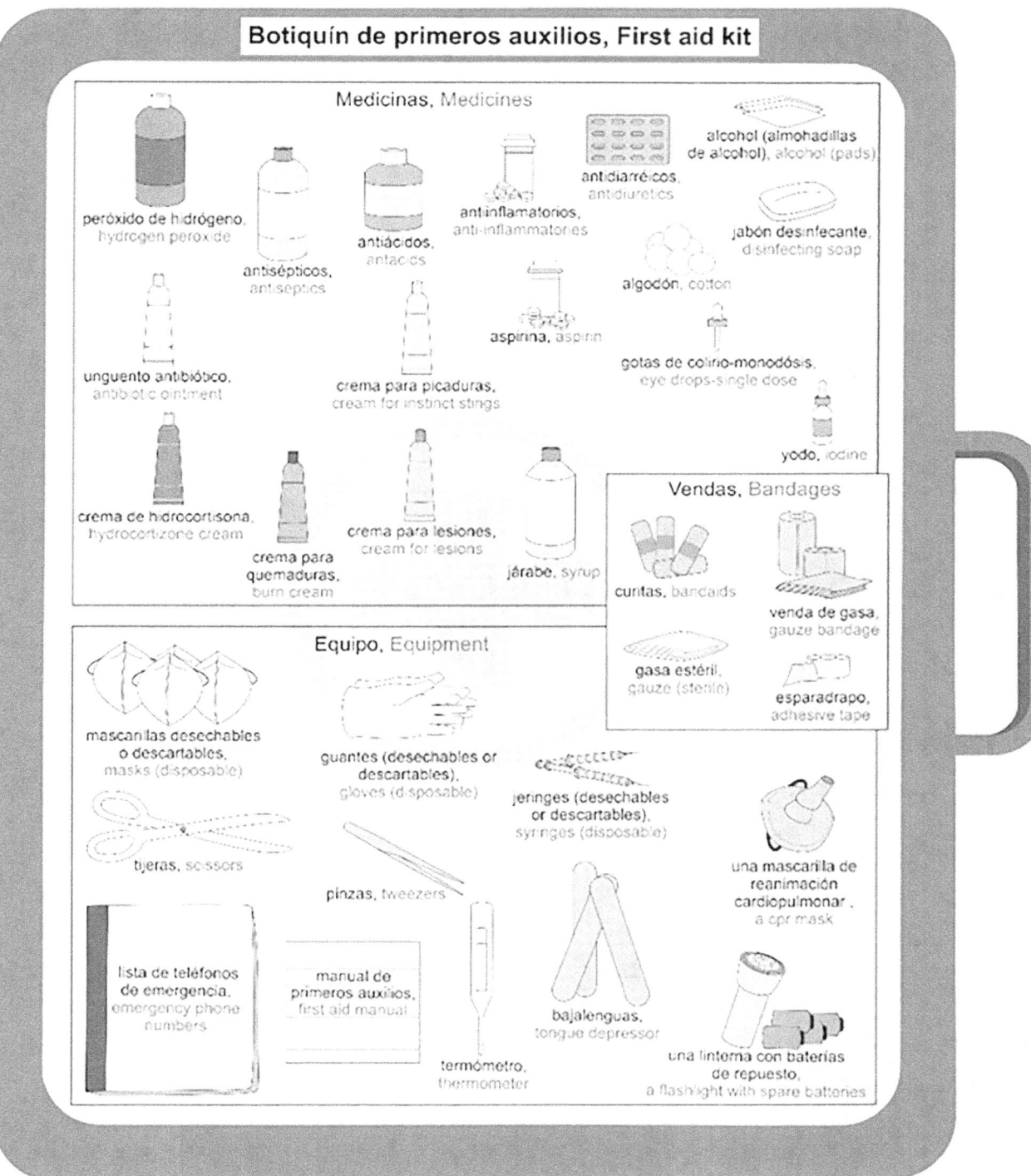

## Botiquín de primeros auxilios, First aid kit

### Medicinas, Medicines

peróxido de hidrógeno, hydrogen peroxide

antisépticos, antiseptics

antiácidos, antacids

anti-inflamatorios, anti-inflammatories

antidiarréicos, antidiuretics

alcohol (almohadillas de alcohol), alcohol (pads)

jabón desinfecante, disinfecting soap

algodón, cotton

aspirina, aspirin

gotas de colirio-monodósis, eye drops-single dose

unguento antibiótico, antibiotic ointment

crema para picaduras, cream for instinct stings

yodo, iodine

crema de hidrocortisona, hydrocortizone cream

crema para quemaduras, burn cream

crema para lesiones, cream for lesions

járabe, syrup

### Vendas, Bandages

curitas, bandaids

venda de gasa, gauze bandage

gasa estéril, gauze (sterile)

esparadrapo, adhesive tape

### Equipo, Equipment

mascarillas desechables o descartables, masks (disposable)

guantes (desechables or descartables), gloves (disposable)

jeringes (desechables or descartables), syringes (disposable)

una mascarilla de reanimación cardiopulmonar, a cpr mask

tijeras, scissors

pinzas, tweezers

lista de teléfonos de emergencia, emergency phone numbers

manual de primeros auxilios, first aid manual

bajalenguas, tongue depressor

termómetro, thermometer

una linterna con baterías de repuesto, a flashlight with spare batteries

# PAIN

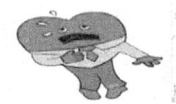 *DOLER* + PAIN EXPRESSIONS

*Doler* is a stem changing *o:ue* verb. Although you can conjugate it in every person, the two most commonly used forms are the third person singular *duele* or the third person plural *duelen*.

The *doler* construction is formed by using an indirect object pronoun (to whom it hurts) + the body part that hurts

HINT: you do not use a possessive to refer to the body part. You use the indefinite article. Possession is expressed in the IDOP (Indirect Object Pronoun).

Ex.
My head hurts. *Me duele la cabeza* or literally *The head hurts me.*
My hands hurt. *Me duelen las manos or literally The hands hurt me.*

| IDOP + duele – | IF ONE BODY PART HURTS |
|---|---|

| IDOP + duelen – | IF MORE THAN ONE BODY PART HURTS |
|---|---|

| Indirect Object Pronoun (IDOP) | |
|---|---|
| Me | *to me* |
| Te | *to you* (familiar) |
| Le | *to him*<br>*to her*<br>*to you* (formal) |
| Nos | *to us* |
| Os | *to you all* (Spain) |
| Les | *to them* or<br>*to you all* (S. America) |

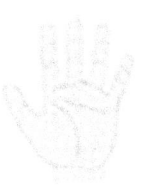 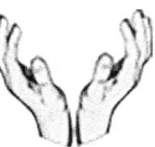

Me/te/le/nos/les duele la mano

Me/te/le/nos/les duelen las manos.

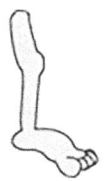

Me/te/le/nos/les duele la naríz

Me/te/le/nos/les duele la pierna

Me/te/le/nos/les duelen las piernas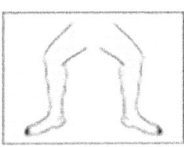

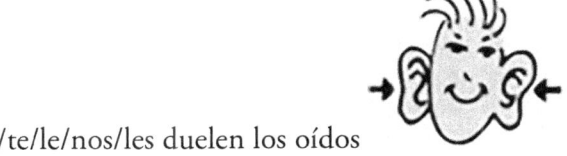

Me/te/le/nos/les duele el oído

Me/te/le/nos/les duelen los oídos

# PAIN ASSESSMENT & TYPES OF PAIN

Patient's Pain Assessment, Evaluación del dolor del paciente

<u>Patient's History of Pain, La historia del dolor del paciente</u>
How long has it hurt you? ¿Cúanto tiempo hace que le duele?
When did the pain start? ¿Cuándo empezó el dolor?
Since when have you had the pain? ¿Desde cuando tiene el dolor?

<u>Patient's Pain Location, El lugar del dolor del paciente</u>
 Where does it hurt? ¿Dónde le duele?
 Point to where it hurts, please. Señale donde le duele, por favor.
 Does it hurt anywhere else? ¿Le duele en otro lugar?
 Does the pain move anywhere? ¿Se traslada el dolor a otro lugar?
Does it hurt when I press here? ¿Le duele cuando le aprieto aquí?
Where does it hurt most?  ¿Dónde le duele más?

Patient's Pain Frequency & Duration, Frecuencia y duración del dolor del paciente

<u>Is the pain… ¿Es el dolor…?</u>
Constant, constante
Comes and goes, va y viene
Every day?, todos los días
How long does the pain last? ¿Cuánto tiempo dura el dolor?

<u>Patient's Type of Pain, El tipo del dolor del paciente</u>
Is the pain …. ¿El dolor es …
light, leve
moderate, moderado
intense, ntenso
severe, severo
unbearable, insoportable

How much does it hurt you? ¿Cuánto le duele?
How much does it hurt on a scale of 1-10?  ¿Cuánto le duele en una escala de uno a diez?
How long does the pain hurt? ¿Cuándo le dura el dolor?

<u>Factors that aggravate or relieve the pain, Los factores que empeoran/ mejoran el dolor</u>
What makes the pain start? ¿Qué hace que su dolor comience?
What makes it hurt less? ¿Qué alivia el dolor?
What makes it hurt more? ¿Qué hace empeorar el dolor?
Is the pain worse when you… ¿Es el dolor peor cuando … ?
    feel stressed? está estresado
    you work? está trabajando
    you sit down? se siente/está sentado
    you get up? se levanta

<u>As Impact of pain on patient, El impacto del dolor al paciente</u>
Does the pain affect….? ¿El dolor afecta …?
your   appetite, … su apetito?
your work, … su trabajo?
your social life, …su vida social?
Has the pain ever affected your sleep? ¿El dolor lo ha despertado de dormir?

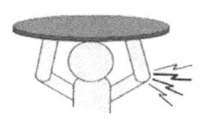
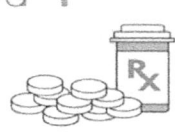

16

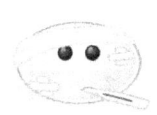 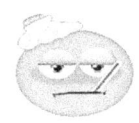

# AILMENTS          DOLENCIAS Y SINTOMAS

| | | | | |
|---|---|---|---|---|
| allergy →la alergía | anemia →la anemia | anxiety →la ansiedad | asthma → el asma | bite →la mordedura |
| blood clot →el coágulo de sangre | broken leg →la pierna rota | bump →la roncha | bruise →el moretón | chicken pox →la varicela |
| chills → los escalofríos | cold →el catarro, el resfriado<br><br>Common cold →el resfriado común | constipated →estreñido,a | Coronavirus →el coronavirus | cramp →el calambre |
| cut →la cortadura | depression → la depresión | diabetes → la diabetes | diarrhea →la diarrea | dry mouth →la boca seca |
| fever→ la fiebre yellow fever→ la fiebre amarilla | flu →la gripe | food poisoning → la intoxicación alimentaria | fracture →la fractura | hay fever → la fiebre del heno |

17

| | | | | |
|---|---|---|---|---|
| high blood pressure/ low blood pressure → la presión arterial alta/baja | hiccups → tener hipo | hemorrhoids → las hemorroides | insect bite → *la picadura de insecto* | insomnia → el insomnio |
| kidney stones →los cálculos renales | laryngitis → la laringitis | lump → el bulto | measles → el sarampión | Migraine →la migraña |
| mouth sores →las úlceras bucales | mumps → las paperas | nose bleed →la hemorragia nasal | palpitations →las palpitaciones | shingles → la culebrilla(herpes zoster ) |
| staggering →el tambaleo | Stomach flu → la gripe estomacal | Stress →el estrés | sun stroke →la insolación | sunburn → la quemadura de sol |
| seizures →los ataques epilépticos | ulcer →la úlcera | vertigo → el vértigo | virus →el virus | wart →la verruga |

18

# SYMPTOMS

| | | | |
|---|---|---|---|
| bleeding →el sangrado to cough up blood-toser sangre | Blurry vision →visión borrosa | Burning (feeling) →el ardor | cough →tos |
| dizzy → mareado  dizzy spells-mareos | *Extreme exhaustion →el cansancio extremo* | faint →el desmayo  To faint→desmayarse | fatigue or weakness  *fatiga o debilidad* |
| heartburn →acidez estomacal or ardor | inflammation →inflamación | irregular heartbeat → el latido irregular del corazón | itching  *picazón/comezón/picor* |
| lack of appetite →la falta de apetito | nausea →náusea | numbness →adormecimiento | Pain →el dolor Headache →el dolor de cabeza Stomach ache →el dolor de estómago |
| rash →sarpullido | redness→el enrojecimiento | shortness of breath → falta de aliento | Sneeze →el estornudo |

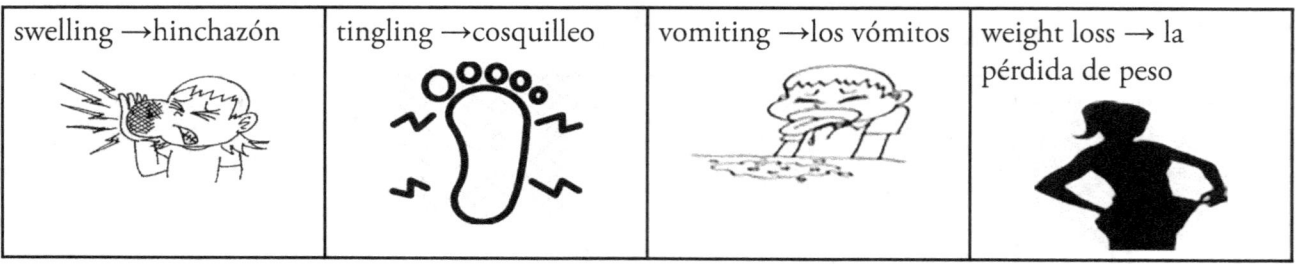

| swelling →hinchazón | tingling →cosquilleo | vomiting →los vómitos | weight loss → la pérdida de peso |

**OJO** *take note* **FOLK ILLNESS**, otherwise referred to as a culture-bound syndrome, or a culture-specific syndrome, is a disease recognizable only by a specific culture or society. Some examples of folk illness or culture-bound syndrome / culture-specific syndroms in Latin America are :*empacho, susto* **or** *mal de susto, nervios, caída de mollera* **and** *mal de ojo*. *Empacho* is a Central American folk illness, referring to gastrointestinal issues. It is characterized by obstruction of the stomach and or intestine. The symptoms of *empacho* include abdominal pain, bloating, nausea, vomiting, lethargy and diarrhea. *Empacho* is believed to be caused by food sticking to the intestinal wall due to eating certain foods at incorrect times, swallowing gum, swallowing too much saliva, among other things. Another folk illness common to Latin American cultures is *susto*. *Susto or mal de susto* can be medically diagnosed as reactive depression or a post-traumatic stress syndrome caused by a traumatic event. Symptoms of *susto* are nervousness, fever, depression, diarrhea and lethargy. Another folk illness similar to *susto* is *nervios*. *Nervios* can consist of trembling, shouting, seizures, fainting spells. *Caída de mollera* refers to "fallen fontanel" and many times is attributed to maternal neglect. The medical diagnosis *of caída de mollera* is dehydration. This is caused by pulling the baby from the breast or bottle too quickly or holding the baby incorrectly or letting the baby fall. A very common Latin American folk-illness is *mal de ojo*. The translation of *mal de ojo* is an 'evil eye'. [From Spanish *mal* illness + *de* of + *ojo* an eye] (Oxford Reference)*Mal de ojo* is common to many Mediterranean countries and Latino communities. *Mal de ojo* is caused by the jealousy or envy of admirers. The symptoms can range from irritability, crying, fever. Common symptoms of *mal de ojo* are insomnia, diarrhea, vomiting and fever.

## GENERAL PAIN EXPRESSIONS

| | | | | |
|---|---|---|---|---|
| It doesn't hurt.<br>No me duele. | It hurts a little.<br>Me duele un poquito. | The pain is unbearable.<br>El dolor es insoportable. | The pain is sharp.<br>El dolor es agudo. | The pain is dull.<br>El dolor es sordo. |
| The pain is chronic.<br><br>El dolor es crónico. | The pain is intense.<br><br>El dolor es intenso. | I have pain that lasts a short duration.<br>Tengo dolor de corta duración. | I have long term pain.<br>Tengo dolor que dura mucho.<br>Tiempo. | It hurts a lot.<br>Me duele mucho. |
| It is pain with pressure.<br>Es dolor con presión. | It is intermittent pain that comes and goes.<br>Es dolor que va y viene (dolor intermitente). | The pain is constant.<br>El dolor es constante. | The pain is throbbing.<br>El dolor es punzante. | The pain is sharp and fleeting.<br>El dolor es agudo y fugaz. |

## PHARMACY VOCABULARY REFERENCE

| | |
|---|---|
| aftershave, | after shave |
| antibiotic , | el antibiótico |
| antihistamines , | los antihistamínicos |
| antiseptic, | el antiséptico |
| aspirin, | la aspirina |
| athlete's foot powder, | polvos para el pie de atleta |
| bandages, | vendas |
| cough mixture, | jarabe para la tos |
| baby foods, | comida para bebé |
| baby wipes, | toallitas para bebés |
| the band aid, | la curita / las tiritas |
| cold medicine, | antigripal |
| comb, | peine |
| conditioner, | acondicionador |
| condoms, | condones |
| contact lens solution, | líquido par alas lentillas |
| contraceptives, | anticonceptivos |
| cotton, | algodón |
| cough syrup, | jarabe para la tos |
| counter assistant | el (la) asistente de la caja registradora |
| cream/gel, | crema/gel /la pomada |
| dental floss, | hilo dental |
| deodorant, | desodorante |
| diapers (disposable diapers), | pañales (pañales desechables) |
| diarrhea tablets, | comprimidos contra la diarrea |
| dispensing assistant | el (la) asistente de dispensación (o despacho) |
| the eyedrop, | el colirio |
| emergency contraception | (también conocida como the morning after pill), anticonceptivo de emergencia (la píldora del día después) |
| emergency pharmacy- | la farmacia de guardia |
| eye drops, | gotas para los ojos |
| eyeliner, | lápiz de ojos |

| | |
|---|---|
| eyeshadow, | sombra de ojos |
| face powder, | maquillaje en polvos |
| first aid kit, | maletín de primeros auxilios ; el botiquín |
| Hairbrush, | el cepillo |
| hair colouring o hair dye, | el tinte para el pelo |
| hair gel gomina, | fijador para el pelo |
| hair spray, | laca |
| hair wax, | cera para el pelo |
| hand cream, | crema de manos |
| hay fever tablets, | comprimidos contra la fiebre del heno |
| hot water bottle, | bolsa de agua caliente |
| Ibuprofen, | ibuprofeno |
| indigestion tablets, | pastillas para la digestión |
| inhaler/pump, | inhalador/bombilla |
| the injectable, | el inyectable |
| laxative, | el laxante |
| lip balm o lip salve, | el protector labial |
| lip gloss, | el brillo de labios |
| lipstick, | el pintalabios |
| make-up, | el maquillaje |
| mascara, | el rímel |
| medicine, | la medicina; el medicamento |
| moisturizing cream, | la crema hidratante |
| mouthwash, | enjuague bucal |
| nail file, | la lima de uñas |
| nail polish, | el esmalte de uñas |
| nail varnish remover, | el quitaesmalte de uñas |
| nail scissors, | tijeras para uñas |
| nicotine patches, | parches de nicotina |
| on-line pharmacy → | la farmacia en línea |
| painkillers, | analgésico |
| paracetamol, | paracetamol |
| panty liners, | salva slip |
| pharmacist, | farmacéutica/o |

| | |
|---|---|
| pharmacy technician | *el (la) técnico(a) de la farmacia* |
| pills, | las pastillas |
| plasters, | esparadrapo |
| pregnancy testing kit, | prueba de embarazo |
| prescription, | receta |
| razor, | maquinilla de afeitar |
| razorblade, | cuchilla de afeitar |
| sanitary towels, | toallitas sanitarias |
| shampoo, | champú |
| shaving brush, | brocha de afeitar |
| shaving cream, | crema para el afeitado |
| shaving foam, | espuma para el afeitado |
| shaving gel, | gel para el afeitado |
| shower gel, | gel de ducha |
| soap, | jabón |
| safety pins, | imperdibles |
| sleeping tablets, | pastillas para dormir |
| sun cream, | crema solar |
| sun block, | el bloqueador solar |
| tampons, | tampones |
| thermometer, | termómetro |
| throat lozenges, | pastillas para el dolor de garganta |
| tissues, | pañuelos de papel |
| travel sickness, tablets | pastillas contra el mareo |
| toothbrush, | cepillo de dientes |
| toothpaste, | pasta de dientes |
| tweezers, | pinzas |
| vitamin pills, | pastillas de vitaminas |

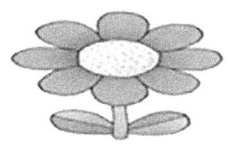

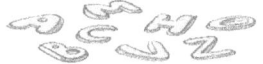

**Alfabeto**

Alphabet in Spanish, El Abecedario (Alfabeto)

| Letter | Letter Name | Pronunciation | Example |
|--------|-------------|---------------|---------|
| A | a | Sounds like the English **ah** | ambulancia |
| B | be (also called be larga, be grande or be de burro) | Often sounds like the English **b.** When between 2 vowels, it is pronounced much like the Spanish **v** (lips not touching) | biopsia |
| C | ce | Sounds like an English **s** if followed by a soft vowel (e or i ). Sounds like an English **k,** if followed by a consonant or a hard vowel (a, o, u) | cirugía   camilla |
| CH | che | Sounds like an English **ch**; no longer considered a letter by RAE | chata |
| D | de | Sounds much like the English **d**. It is usually a softer sound, like **th** in English, especially when between 2 vowels | doctor |
| E | e | Sounds like **eh** in English | emergencia |
| F | efe | Sounds like an English **f** | fiebre |
| G | ge | Sounds like an English **g,** if  followed by a consonant or a hard vowel (a, o,u); sounds like a harsh h if followed by a soft vowel (e or i ). | ginecólogo   gaza |
| H | hache | As a general rule, this letter is silent if it is the first letter of a word. The exception to this rule are words adopted from other languages, which maintain the breathy aspiration, such as Hawáii. | hospital |
| I | I | Sounds like **ee** in English, but shorter | insulina |
| J | jota | Sounds like **h** in English | jeringa |
| K | ca | Sounds like **k** in English. The letter K is not native to the Spanish language & only appears in loanwords such as karate, kilo | kilómetro |
| L | ele | Sounds like the English **l,** (tongue raised closer to the roof of the mouth; not dipped) | laringitis |
| LL | doble ele | Sounds like 'y' in English (no longer considered a letter by RAE) | llaga |

25

| | | | |
|---|---|---|---|
| M | eme | Sounds like the English *m* | mamografía |
| N | ene | Sounds like the English *n* | neurología |
| Ñ | eñe | Sounds like the *ni* in onion or the *ny* in canyon | riñon |
| O | o | Sounds like the *o* in *so*, but shorter | operación |
| P | pe | Sounds like an English *p* | paperas |
| Q | cu | Always followed by a *u* and sounds like the English *k* | quemadura |
| R | erre | Sounds like the English *r*, but is rolled | rodilla |
| RR | doble erre | Trilled *rr* sound. No longer considered a letter by the RAE | socorro HELP! |
| S | ese | Sounds like an English *s* | sarampión |
| T | te | Sounds like an English *t* *but softer* | tos |
| U | u | Sounds like *oo* in *food* (note that when u is part of dipthong such as ua or ue, it sounds like an English *W*) | urólogo |
| V | ve or uve; also called ve corta, ve chica, ve de vaca | Sounds like the Spanish *b* (The lips don't touch and there is less aspiration) | vacuna |
| W | doble ve or uve doble | The letter *W* is not native to the Spanish language, but sounds like the English *w* & only appears in loanwords such as web & watt | síndrome de Down's |
| X | equis | Sounds like *ks* in English 'socks' | rayo X |
| Y | ye; also called I griega | Sounds like the *y* in English *yes*. At the end of a words, it sounds like the letter *I (hay)* | yodo |
| Z | zeta | Sounds like the Englsih *s;* in many parts of Spain it is a *th* sound | zumbido |

La Real Academia Española (RAE) or Royal Spanish Academy states that the Spanish alphabet has 27 letters. The Spanish language coincides with the English alphabet except that the Spanish alphabet has one additional letter, ñ (In 2010 RAE eliminated CH and LL as letters in Spanish alphabet).

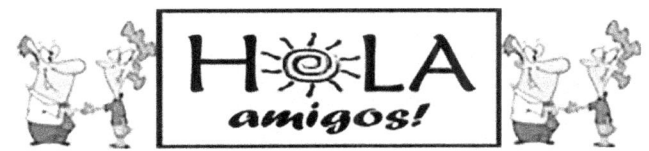

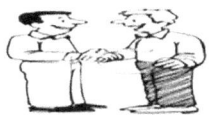

| Greetings & Good-byes | Saludos y despedidas |
|---|---|
| Hello | Hola |
| Good morning | Buenos días |
| Good afternoon | Buenas tardes |
| Good evening | Buenas noches |
| Until... | Hasta + specific future time frame |
| | Example: Until next week. Hasta la semana próxima. |
| See you later | Hasta luego |
| See you tomorrow | Hasta mañana |
| See you soon | Hasta pronto or Hasta la vista |
| Have a nice day | Que tenga un buen día |
| Goodbye | Adiós/ Chau |

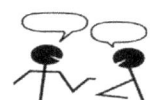

| Basic Daily Expressions | Expresiones diarias |
|---|---|
| What's happening? | ¿ Qué tal? ¿Qué pasa? |
| What's new? What's up? | ¿Qué hay de nuevo? |
| How's it going? (formal) | ¿Cómo le va? |
| How's it going? (familiar) | ¿Cómo te va? |

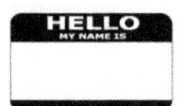

**Name**

What is your  name/ last name? (formal)

What is your  name/ last name? (familiar)

**Introductions**

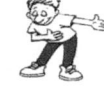

**Introducing yourself**

My name is …

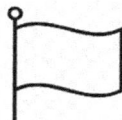

**Introducing Others**

I would like to introduce you to....

Nice to meet you.

It's a pleasure to meet you. (formal)

It's a pleasure to meet you. (familiar)

My pleasure.

Charmed.

**Nationality**

Where are you from ? (formal)

Where are you from ?   (familiar)

I am from_____.

**Nombre**

¿Cómo se llama?

¿Cuál es  su nombre/apellido?

¿Cómo te llamas? ¿Cuál es tu nombre/apellido?

**Presentaciones**

Me llamo _____

Yo soy _____

Mi nombre es  _____

Le presento a...(formal)

Te presento a.. (familiar)

Mucho gusto.

Es un placer conocerle.

Es un placer conocerte.

El placer es mío.

Encantado/a

**Nacionalidad**

¿De dónde es Usted?

¿De dónde eres tú?

Yo soy de_____.(country)

Yo soy_____(nationality)

OJO *take note* : Rules of Thumb for expressing nationality:

Countries are capitalized. Nationalities are not capitalized.

Example: I am from Mexico. Yo soy de México. I am Mexican. Yo soy mexicano/a.

Adjectives of nationality must agree in gender and number with the noun they are referring to. They come after the noun. Example: la comida española (the Spanish food), el restaurante italiano (the Italian restaurant).

The typical endings for adjectives of nationality in Spanish are: *-ano, -ense, -l, -és, -eño,* and *-o.* If the nationality ending is a consonant, add an –a for the feminine version.

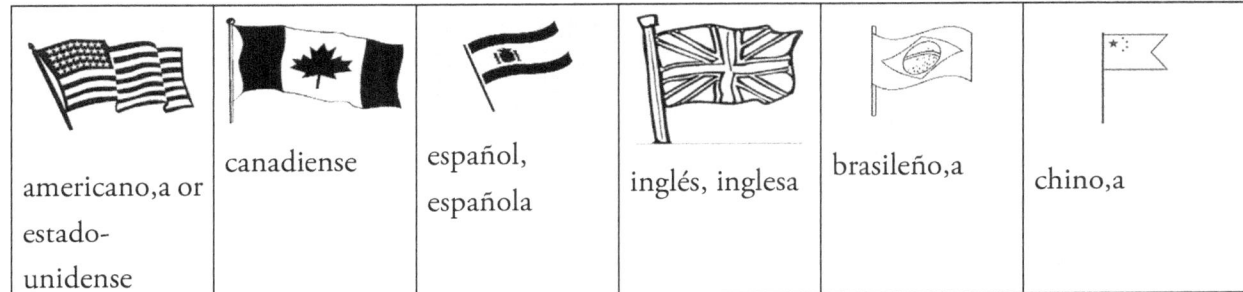

| americano,a or estado-unidense | canadiense | español, española | inglés, inglesa | brasileño,a | chino,a |
|---|---|---|---|---|---|

**Address**

**Dirección**

Where do you live? (formal)

¿Dónde vive Usted?

Where do you live? (familiar)

¿Dónde vives?

I live in_____

Yo vivo en _____

**Profession/Job**

**Profesión / trabajo**

What do you do? (formal)

*¿En qué trabaja? ¿En qué se dedica?*

What do you do? (familiar)

*¿En qué trabajas? ¿En qué te dedicas?*

I am a _____

Yo soy _____

**OJO** *take note* **:** To express someone's line of work use: *SER + occupation or job.* The article is omitted, unless you are adding an adjective to describe the person.

Example: I am a doctor. Yo soy médico,a. I am a kind doctor. Yo soy un médico amable.

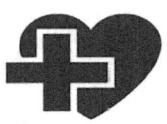

| | |
|---|---|
| **Health** | **Salud** |
| How are you? (formal) | ¿Cómo está Usted? |
| How are you? (familiar) | ¿Cómo estás tú? |
| I am well .. sick ..regular ..so so | Estoy bien..enfermo(a) ....regular..así así |

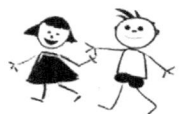

| | |
|---|---|
| **Looks & Personality Traits** | **Razcos físicos y razcos de la personalidad** |
| What are you like? (formal) | ¿Cómo es Usted? |
| What are you like? (familiar) | ¿Cómo eres tú? |
| I am _____ | Yo soy _____ |

**OJO** *take note* **:** Use the verb **ser** to describe essential qualities or intrinsic characteristics of a person or a thing, such as physical appearance and personality traits.

Example: Juan is tall, handsome and nice. Juan es alto, guapo y simpático.

Ana is blond, pretty and hard-working. Ana es rubia, bonita y trabajadora.

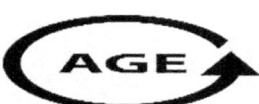

| | |
|---|---|
| **Age** | **Edad** |
| How old are you? | ¿Cúantos años tiene Usted? (formal) |
| | ¿Cúantos años tienes tú ? (familiar) |
| I am _____old. | Yo tengo ___años |

**OJO** *take note* : Age is expressed with the verb **tener** in Spanish. It is one of the many idiomatic expressions with tener. Example: I am 20 years old. Yo tengo veinte años.

| **Expressions of Courtesy** | *Expresiones de cortesía* |
|---|---|
| Thank you | Gracias |
| Please | Por favor |
| You're welcome. | De nada |
| I'm sorry. | Lo siento. |
| Pardon me. | Perdón |
| Excuse me. | Disculpe. Con permiso. |
| Take care. | Cuídese (formal) Cuídate (familiar). |
| Bless you! | (after someone sneezes)¡Salud! |
| Welcome! | ¡Bienvenido(a)! |

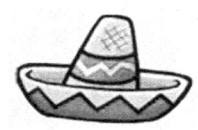

**Days of the week**　　　　　　　**Los días de la semana**

OJO *take note* Days of the week in Spanish are lower case, masculine and are not pluralized except for Saturday & Sunday. The first day of the week is Monday.

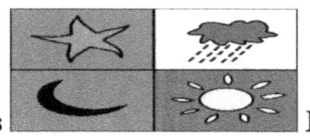

**Seasons & Months**　　　　　　　**Estaciones y meses**

| | | | |
|---|---|---|---|
| Fall → otoño<br>September → el septiembre<br>October → el octubre<br>November → el noviembre | Winter → invierno<br>December → el diciembre<br>January → el enero<br>February → el febrero | Spring → primavera<br>March → el marzo<br>April → el abril<br>May → el mayo | Summer → verano<br>June → el junio<br>July → el julio<br>August-el agosto |

OJO *take note* **To express that an action that is being done on a certain day of the week use 'el' example. Yo trabajo el lunes. I work this Monday. To express an action that is repeated use 'los'. Example: Yo trabajo los lunes. I work every Monday.**

## NUMBERS IN SPANISH:

| Cero<br>**0** | Uno<br>**1** | Dos<br>**2** | Tres<br>**3** | Cuatro<br>**4** | Cinco<br>**5** | Seis<br>**6** |
|---|---|---|---|---|---|---|
| Siete<br>**7** | Ocho<br>**8** | Nueve<br>**9** | Diez<br>**10** | Once<br>**11** | Doce<br>**12** | Trece<br>**13** |
| Catorce<br>**14** | Quince<br>**15** | Diez y seis or<br>Dieciseis<br>**16** | Diez y siete<br>or diecisiete<br>**17** | Diez y ocho<br>or dieciocho<br>**18** | Diez y nueve<br>or diecinueve<br>**19** | Veinte<br>**20** |

OJO *take note* : Add the word 'y' to form any numbers past 30. Example: 35 students Treinta y cinco estudiantes.

| Thirty-treinta | Forty-cuarenta | Fifty –cincuenta | Sixty-sesenta | Seventy-setenta | Eighty-ochenta | Ninety –noventa | One hundred -cien, ciento |
|---|---|---|---|---|---|---|---|
| **30** | **40** | **50** | **60** | **70** | **80** | **90** | **100** |

OJO *take note* Numbers in Spanish precede the noun as in English.

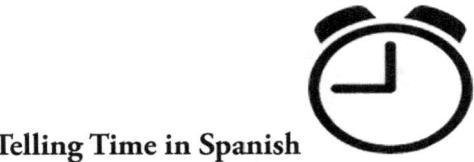

**Telling Time in Spanish**

What time is it?        ¿Qué hora es?

OJO *take note* : ¿Qué hora es? Literally means What hour is it? When telling time in Spanish, the word hour (hora) is implied.

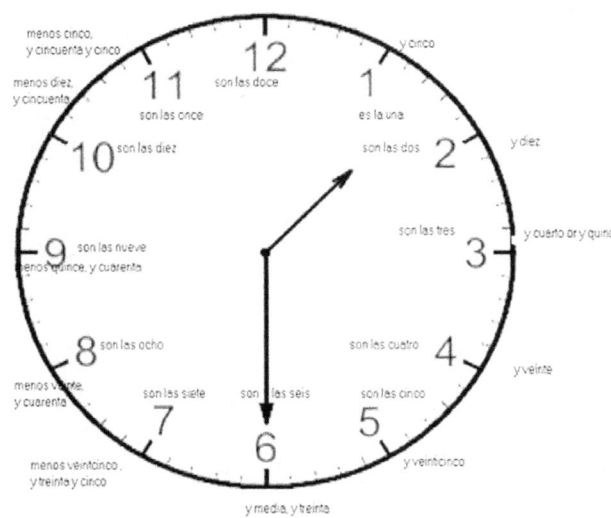

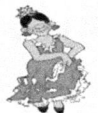

**To tell time:**

**Es la** _____ Use for 1:oo o'clock. Example: It is 1:00. Es la una.

**Son las** _____ Use for any hour greater than 1:00. Example: It is 8:00. Son las ocho.

**OJO** *take note* : The feminine article (*la/las*) is used before the number because it refers to *la hora*.

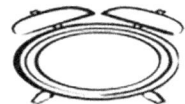 **KEY TIME WORDS:**

Use 'y' (and) to add minutes.

Use 'menos' (less) to subtract minutes.

Use 'en punto' to express 'on the dot'.

Use 'cuarto' or 'quince' to express 15 minutes.

Use 'media' to express half an hour.

Use 'de la mañana' to express AM.

Use 'de la tarde' to express afternoon.

Use 'de la noche' to express PM.

To express time of day use:

- *mediodía* – midday
- *mañana* – in the morning
- *noche* – at night
- *madrugada* – the middle of the night
- *medianoche* – midnight
- *amanecer* – dawn
- *tarde* – in the afternoon

**Seasons**

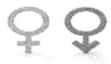 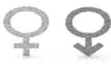

# GENDER & NOUNS IN SPANISH

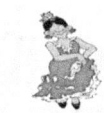

Every noun in Spanish is either masculine or feminine.

## BASIC GENDER RULES

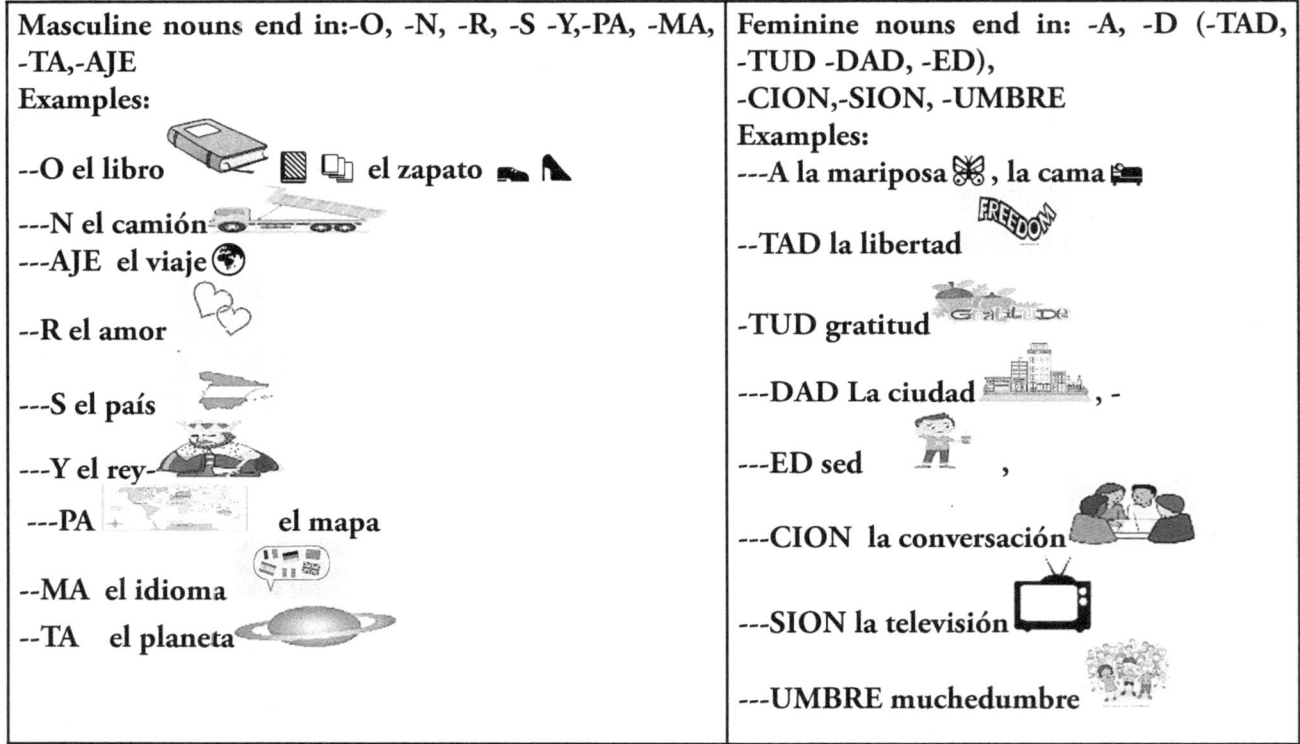

| Masculine nouns end in:-O, -N, -R, -S -Y,-PA, -MA, -TA,-AJE<br>Examples:<br>--O el libro   el zapato<br>---N el camión<br>---AJE el viaje<br>--R el amor<br>---S el país<br>---Y el rey<br>---PA el mapa<br>--MA el idioma<br>--TA el planeta | Feminine nouns end in: -A, -D (-TAD, -TUD -DAD, -ED),<br>-CION,-SION, -UMBRE<br>Examples:<br>---A la mariposa , la cama<br>--TAD la libertad<br>-TUD gratitud<br>---DAD La ciudad , -<br>---ED sed ,<br>---CION la conversación<br>---SION la televisión<br>---UMBRE muchedumbre |

Additional Gender Rules:

♀♀ People or living creatures are referred to by the gender they represent. Example:el chico la chica

♀♀ Mixed gender- If you are referring to a group of people with mixed gender, you must always use the masculine, even if the ratio of males is less than the ratio of females. Example: los niños

♀♀ Nouns ending in -e and referring to a person can be either masculine or feminine. The article changes depending on the gender of the person, but the noun stays the same. Example: el estudiante la estudiante

♀♀ Nouns that end in *-ista* can be both masculine or feminine.  Only the article changes depending on to the gender. Example:

*el turista* –the male turist        *la turista – the female tourist*

*el dentist*-the male dentist        *la dentist*-the female dentist

♀♀ If a masculine noun ends in a consonant, it would have a corresponding female form ending in an *a*.

*Example: el profesor* → the male professor        *la profesora* → the female professor

♀♀ An article can change the meaning of a word. Example: el cura-the priest        la cura-the cure

♀♀ Letters of the alphabet are feminine. Days of the week are masculine.

♀♀ **GENDER TRAP:**. Nouns that do not refer to living creatures follow basic gender rules, regardless of whether they are typically associated with males or females. Example: el vestido 👗  la corbata 👔

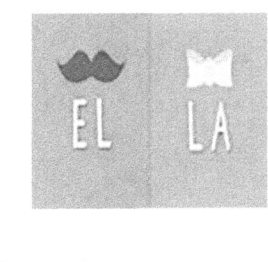

Feminine
Articles

DEFINITE: la, las
INDEFINITE: una, unas

Masculine
Articles
DEFINITE: el, los
INDEFINITE: un, unos

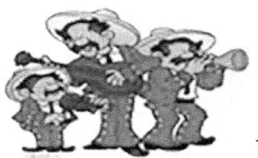

## PLURALS IN SPANISH

| IF A NOUN ENDS IN A VOWEL: **ADD –S** | IF A NOUN ENDS IN A CONSONANT: **ADD –ES** |
|---|---|
| IF A NOUN ENDS IN A –Z: **CHANGE TO -CES** | OJO *take note* if a noun is plural, the adjective following it and the article preceding it must also be plurals |

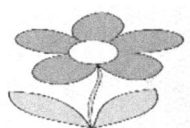

## POSSESSIVES IN SPANISH

**Possessive adjectives in Spanish go before a noun, as in English. In Spanish, possessives agree in number with the noun. The nosotros and vosotros forms also agree in gender.**

| PRONOUN | singular | plural | examples |
|---|---|---|---|
| my | mi | mis | mi sombrero 👒 my hats, mis sombreros 👒 👒 |
| your (familiar) | Tu | tus | tu casa 🏠 tus casas 🏠 🏠 |
| his, hers, your (formal), its | su | sus | su bicicleta 🚲 sus bicicletas 🚲 🚲 |
| our | nuestro, nuestra | nuestros, nuestras | nuestra manzana 🍎 nuestras manzanas 🍎 🍎 nuestro helado 🍦, nuestros helados 🍦 🍦 |
| your (all) Spain | Vuestro, vuestra | Vuestros, vuestras | vuestra cuchara 🥄 vuestras cucharas 🥄 🥄 |
| Their , your (all) Latin America | su | sus | su hamburguesa 🍔 , sus hammburguesas 🍔 🍔 |

OJO *take note* 'Su' and 'sus' can mean his, hers, yours (formal) its, their or your (plural-Latin America). 'Su' should always be used when the noun is singular and 'sus' should always be used when the noun is plural. example: su casa or sus casas.

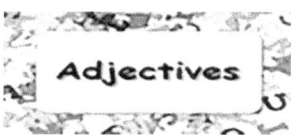

OJO *take note* Adjectives agree in gender and number with the noun they modify.

| angry<br><br>ENOJADO (A)<br><br>Enojado/a/os/as | Happy<br><br>Feliz/felices or<br>Contento/a/os/as | Bored<br><br>Aburrido/a/os/as | Nice<br><br>Simpático/a/os/as |
|---|---|---|---|
| Mean/nasty<br><br>Antipático/a/os/as | Smart<br><br>Inteligente/s | Beatiful-lindo/a/os/as<br><br>Pretty-bonito/a/os/as | Handsome<br><br>Guapo/a/o/os |
| Ugly<br><br>Feo/a/os/as | Fat<br><br>Gordo/a/os/as | Skinny<br><br>Delgado/a/os/as | Tall<br><br>Alto/a/os/as |

OJO *take note* : The rule of thumb regarding placement of nouns and adjectives is **QUANTITY BEFORE QUALITY.**

Example: Ten intelligent nurses would be Diez enfermeras/os inteligentes. Adjectives follow the noun that they modify and agree in gender & in number with the noun that they modify.

39

**Demonstrative Adjectives**-denote distance of an object or person in relation to the speaker

| Distance from speaker | Masculine singular | Masculine plural | Feminine singular | Feminine plural |
|---|---|---|---|---|
| Close-this & these | **este** | **estos** | **esta** | **estas** |
| farther -that & those | **ese** | **esos** | **esa** | **esas** |
| Farthest-that & those | **aquel** | **aquellos** | **aquella** | **aquellas** |

OJO *take note* : If the noun **is not identified**, is **abstract, or is unknown**, the *neuter demonstrative pronouns* **esto, eso**, and **aquello** are used.

Examples:  Este libro. This book  (CLOSEST TO THE SPEAKER)

Ese libro. That book. (FURTHER FROM THE SPEAKER)

**Aquel libro. That book over there.  (FURTHEST FROM THE SPEAKER)**

OJO *take note* : **EASY WAY TO REMEMBER: this & these have the 't's**

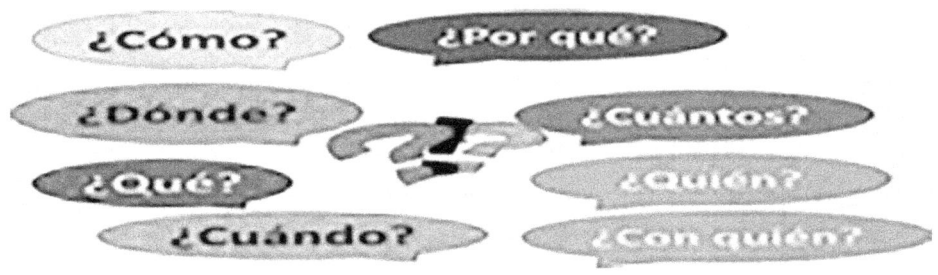

| 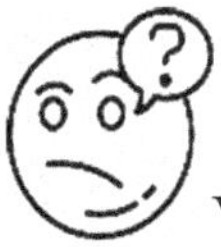 | WHERE | HOW | WHAT/WHICH |
|---|---|---|---|
| WHO | DONDE-location | COMO | QUE |
| QUIEN (singular) | | ¿Cómo se llama? | ¿Qué hora es? |
| QUIENES (plural) | ¿Dónde vives? | | ¿A qué hora es la clase? |
| TO WHOM | A DONDE-destination | | |
| A QUIEN (singular) | | | |
| A QUIENES (plural) | ¿A dónde vas? | | |
| WITH WHOM | DE DONDE-nationality | | |
| CON QUIEN (singular) | ¿De dónde eres? | | |
| CON QUIENES (plural) | | | |
| FOR WHOM | | | |
| PARA QUIEN (singular) | | | |
| PARA QUIENES (plural) | | | |
| WHOSE-possession | | | |
| DE QUIEN (singular) | | | |
| DE QUIENES (plural) | | | |
| ¿Quién es su cantante favorito? | | | |
| ¿Quiénes son sus amigos? | | | |

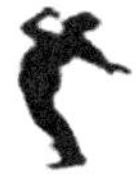

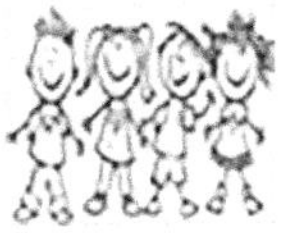

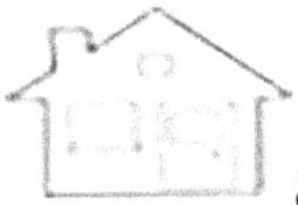

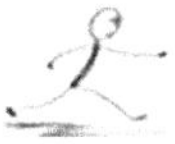

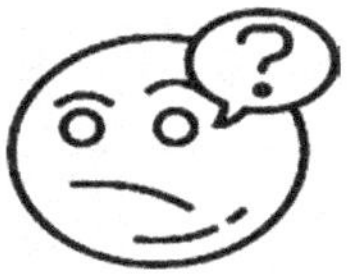

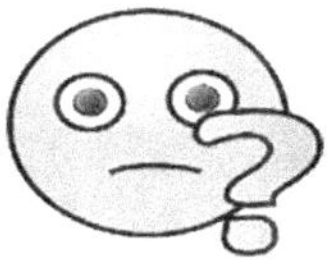

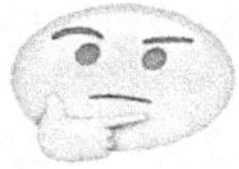

| HOW MUCH/HOW MANY CUANTO, A<br>¿Cuánto cuesta?<br>**CUANTOS, AS**<br>¿Cuántos estudiantes hay en la clase? | WHY<br>**PORQUE** 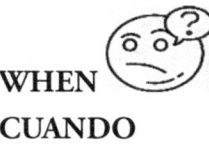<br>¿Por qúe estás triste? | WHEN<br>**CUANDO** 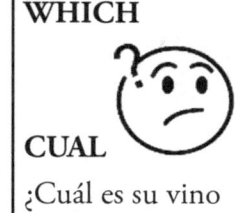<br>¿Cuándo es el concierto? | WHICH<br>**CUAL**<br>¿Cuál es su vino favorito? |
| --- | --- | --- | --- |

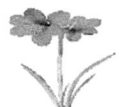

## SPANISH PRONOUN CHART

**OJO** *take note* Pronouns are key to mastering Spanish grammar. Below are 4 **MUST KNOW** types of pronouns in Spanish:

| Subject pronouns | Reflexive Pronouns | DOP | IDOP |
| --- | --- | --- | --- |
| Yo-I | me | me | me |
| Tú (you familiar) | te | te | te |
| Él, ella, Usted | se | lo, la | le |
| nosotros | nos | nos | nos |
| vosotros | os | os | os |
| Ellos, ellas, Uds | se | los,las | les |

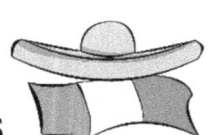

## SUBJECT PRONOUNS

**OJO** *take note* **In Spanish, subject pronouns are generally used for** emphasis or clarity. Unlike in English, in Spanish you can omit a personal pronoun before a verb. The verb conjugations make clear the subject of the sentence. For example: **Hablas español.** *You speak Spanish.* **Hablamos español.** *We speak Spanish.* The 3rd person singular or plural is where there is room for ambiguity because the 3rd person singular can be he, she, you (formal) or it.

OJO *take note* **There is no equivalent translation for the subject pronoun "it" . You simply omit the subject pronoun altogether and use the 3rd person of the verb: Es bonita.** *It is beautiful.* **Funciona bien.** *It works well.*

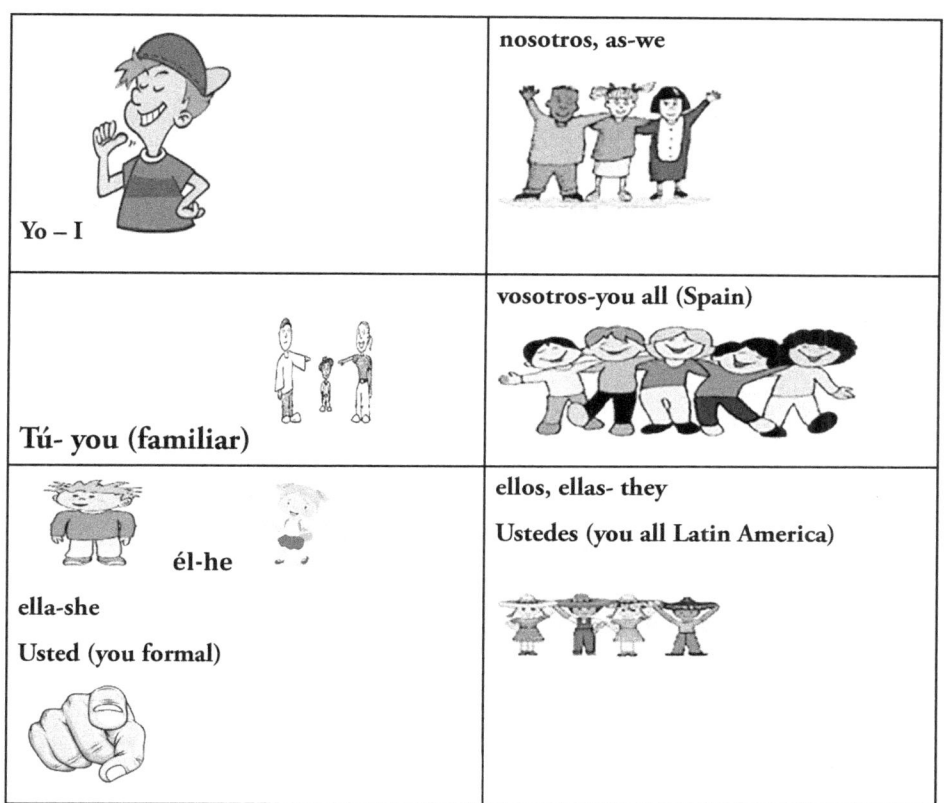

OJO *take note* **In Spanish there are two personal pronouns for** *"you"* **singular: tú and usted.**

**Tú** is used informally, i.e when talking to a friend, a person we know well, a child, young people and someone that you would address on a first-name basis.

**Usted** is used formally, i.e when talking to a person you do not know, someone who is older, or someone you are addressing with a title.

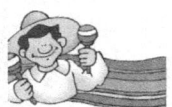

## Reflexive Pronouns

OJO *take note* Reflexive verbs reflect back to the person doing the action. They are used only if the subject is doing the action to themselves.

The verb 'lavar' is an example of this concept. It can be used as lavar (non-reflexive) or lavarse (reflexive). The key is who is the subject doing the action to.

Example: I wash the car. Yo lavo el coche. (the subject does the action to the car) Juan washes the pet. Juan lava el mascote. (the subject does the action to the pet) Therefore, no reflexive is needed.

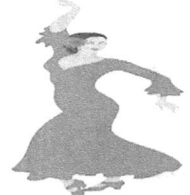

**NON REFLEXIVE**                    **REFLEXIVE**

| Yo lavo | Nosotros lavamos | Yo me lavo | Nosotros nos lavamos |
|---|---|---|---|
| Tú lavas | Vosotros laváis | Tú te lavas | Vosotros os laváis |
| Él, ella, Ud lava | Ellos, ellas, Uds lavan | Él, ella, Usted Se lava | Ellos, ellas, Uds Se lavan |

EXAMPLES: I wash myself. Me lavo. Juan washes himself. Juan se lava. We wash ourselves. Nos lavamos. (The subject does the action to themselves).

OJO *take note* Some common reflexive verbs in Spanish are daily routine verbs such as despertarse (to wake up), bañarse- to take a bath, ducharse-to take a shower, maquillarse-to put on makeup, afeitarse- to shave.

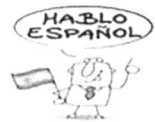

## Direct & Indirect Object Pronouns

OJO *take note*    To figure out which is the direct object and which is the indirect object of a sentence, your starting point is always the **subject and verb of the sentence.**

DOP (Direct Object Pronoun) –Answers the question '**who or what**' with regard to the verb. A DOP can be a person, place or thing. Ex. I read <u>the book.</u> I read it. Julia loves <u>Miguel.</u> Julia loves him

### DOP Rules of Thumb:

In English the order is verb +DOP. In Spanish the order is DOP + verb for simple sentences (the rule changes when you have 2 verbs together)

Example: Juan lee <u>el libro.</u> Juan **lo** lee. Juan reads the book. Juan reads it.

IDOP (Indirect Object Pronoun)-Aswers the question '**to whom, for whom**' with regard to the verb and is usually found at the end of the sentence. IDOPs always refer to a person. Example: Jorge buys the book <u>for Juan.</u> Jorge buys the book for him.

### IDOP Rules of Thumb:

In English the order is verb + IDOP. In Spanish, the order is IDOP + verb. (the rule changes when you have 2 verbs together)

Example: Juan reads the book to Geraldo. Juan **le** lee el libro.

OJO *take note*  The 3rd person 'le' can mean to him, to her, to you (formal) or to it (such as a pet). You can use context to figure out who it is referring to or you add a clarifier to a sentence Example-Yo le doy la computadora a Jorge. The clarifier ' a Jorge', lets the reader know that 'le' in this case, is to him or to Jorge.

**Direct & Indirect Object Pronouns TOGETHER**

In Spanish, as in English, you can use both DOPs & IDOPs in a sentence together .

**DOP & IDOP TOGETHER Rules of Thumb:**

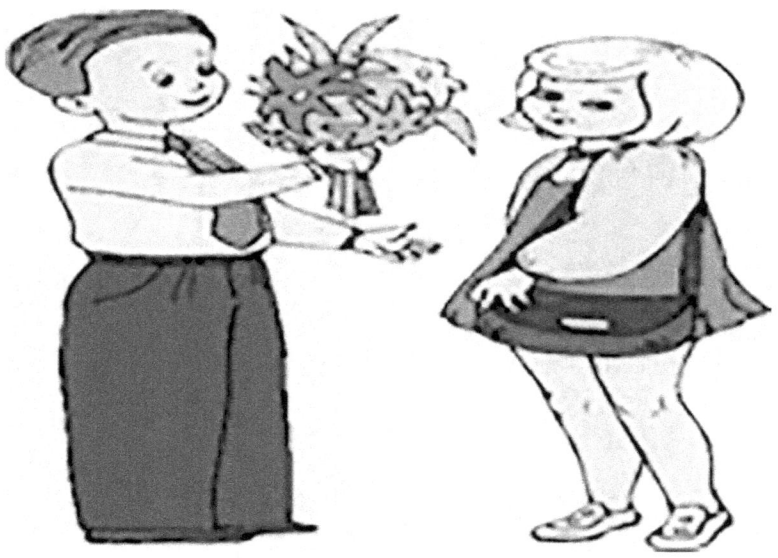

SPANISH: IDOP + DOP + verb (English: verb + DOP + IDOP)

DOP-answers the question 'what or who'

IDOP-answers the question 'to whom'

Juan gives flowers to me. Juan gives them to me.

Juan da las flores a mí. Juan me las da.

OJO *take note* In English, the order for IDOP & DOPs used together is verb+DOP+IDOP .
In Spanish the order is IDOP+DOP+verb for simple sentences (the rule changes when you have 2 verbs
together).

Example. I read the book to you (familiar). I read it to you. Yo **te lo** leo.

OJO *take note* In Spanish you can never have an indirect and direct object that both start with an 'l'. You must substitute the indirect object with the pronoun 'se'. Example- Yo doy el libro a Juan. Yo le lo doy is incorrect. You must say: Yo se lo doy.

SPANISH: IDOP + DOP + verb (English: verb + DOP + IDOP)

DOP-answers the question 'what or who'

IDOP-answers the question 'to whom'

Juan gives flowers to Marta. Juan gives them to her.

Juan da las flores a Marta.  Juan le las da IS INCORRECT. 'LE' becomes 'SE'. CORRECT ANSWER: Juan se las da.

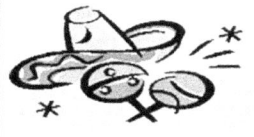

**VERBS –In Spanish there are 3 types of verbs: -ar, -er, -ir**

**REGULAR VERB ENDINGS FOR –AR, -ER & -IR VERBS**

OJO *take note* The subject or subject pronoun determines which ending to use.

| Subject Pronoun | Habl-ar | Com-er | Viv-ir |
|---|---|---|---|
| Yo | Habl-o | Com-o | Viv-o |

| Tú | Habl-as | Com-es | Viv-es |
| Él, ella, Usted | Habl-a | Com-e | Viv-e |
| Nosotros | Habl-amos | Com-emos | Viv-imos |
| Vosotros | Habl-áis | Com-éis | Viv-ís |
| Ellos, ellas, Ustedes | Habl-an | Com-en | Viv-en |

**OJO** ( 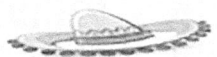 Vosotros (you all-addressing a group of people)is used in Spain and Ustedes (you all-plural), is used in Latin America. You may hear a variation of vosotros in Argentina or Colombia, ex -Vos trabajás (you work).

**SER VS ESTAR –In Spanish, there are two verbs that mean 'to be'.**

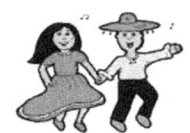

SER                                                                 ESTAR

| Yo soy | Yo estoy |
| Tú eres | Tú estás |
| Él, ella, Usted es | Él, ella, Usted está |
| Nosotros somos | Nosotros estamos |
| Ellos,ellas, Ustedes son | Ellos,ellas, Ustedes estan |

| ESTAR-used for temporary, or changeable situations (acronym-HELP) | SER-used for situations considered permanent-(acronym DOCTOR) |
| H= health | DATE |

48

| | |
|---|---|
| E = emotions or mood<br><br>☺ contento/a or feliz ☹ triste,<br>😠 enojado/a aburrido/a 😐 | OCCUPATION |
| L=location | CHARACTERISTIC (looks or intrinsic characteristic) |
| P=present progressive USE ESTAR TO FORM THE PRESENT PROGRESSIVE<br>ESTAR + ando for –ar verbs<br>ESTAR + -iendo for –er & -ir verbs | TIME |
| or present temporary condition | ORIGIN (NATIONALITY) |
| | RELATION (Relationships to someone, what something is made of & possesion or ownership) |

OJO take note Ser & estar both have different uses .They can not be interchanged without affecting the meaning.

| | |
|---|---|
| To be boring- Ser aburrido/a | To be bored -Estar aburrido/a |
| To be clever -Ser listo/a | To be ready- Estar listo/a<br>Ready |

49

| | |
|---|---|
| To be conceited -Ser orgulloso/a | To be proud- Estar orgulloso/a |
| To be rich -Ser rico/a | To be tasty- Estar rico/a |
| To be safe- Ser seguro/a | To be certain -Estar seguro/a |
| To be bad- Ser malo | To be ill- Estar malo |

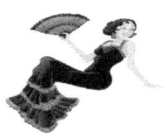

# PREPOSITIONS OF LOCATION

| | | | |
|---|---|---|---|
| *In front of*<br>*Enfrente de, delante de*<br><br>Los libros están delante del chico. | *Next to*<br>*Al lado de*<br><br>El perro está al lado del hombre. | To the left<br>*A la izquierda de*<br><br>La niña está sentada a la izquierda del pupitre. | To the right<br>*A la derecha de*<br><br>La niña está sentada a la derecha del pupitre. |
| Under    *debajo de*<br><br>*La pelota está debajo de la mesa* | *Around*<br>*Alrededor de*<br>La familia está alrededor de la mesa. | *On/upon*<br>*Sobre*<br>Los libros están sobre la mesa. | Between<br>*Entre*<br>El plato está entre la cuchara y el tenedor. |
| Inside dentro de<br><br>El niño está dento de la caja. | Behind<br>*Detrás de*<br><br>La pizarra está detrás del profesor. | Close to - *Cerca de*<br><br>El hombre está cerca de la mujer. | Far from<br>*Lejos de*<br><br>El chico está lejos de la casa. |

OJO *take note* **Prepositions of location are used with the verb estar**

**IRREGULAR VERBS IN SPANISH**  **VERBOS IRREGULARES**

| **IR – to go** | OJO *take note* IR + A + INFINITIVE is a future construction used toexpress a future action.<br>Ex- Voy a trabajar. I am going to work |
|---|---|
| Yo voy | Nosotros vamos |
| Tú vas | Vosotros vaís |
| Él, ella, Ud va | Ellos, ellas, Ustedes van |
| **TENER-to have** | OJO: *take note* Tener has many idiomatic expressions such as : Tener frío-to be cold, tener calor-to be hot, tener __ años-to be ____ years old<br>Tener + que+ INFINITIVE= To have to do something |
| Yo tengo | Nosotros tenemos |
| Tú tienes | Vosotros tenéis |
| Él, ella, Usted tiene | Ellos, ellas, Ustedes tienen |

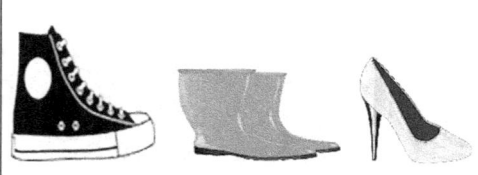

**STEM CHANGING VERBS** -also referred to as SHOE, BOOT, SNEAKER VERBS.
There are 4 different types: **o:ue, e:ie, e:i, u:ue (jugar-to play-is the only u:ue stem-changing verb).**

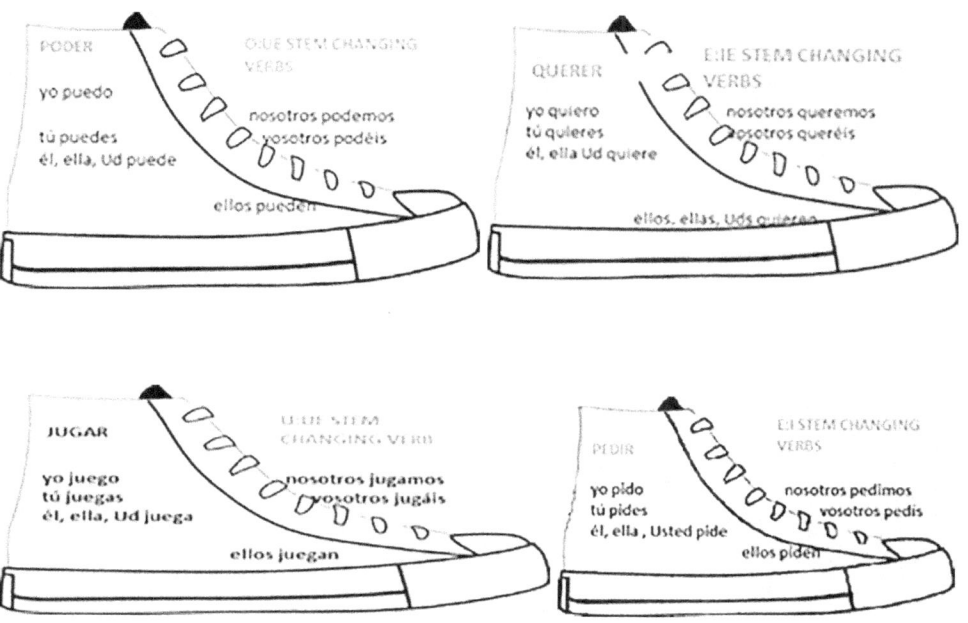

OJO *take note* **The stem**-changing verbs are classified as shoe/boot/sneaker verbs to facilitate learning their conjugations for the beginner student. Shoe verbs have stem changes in every form except nosotros & vosotros. They are classified as shoe verbs because both nosotros & vosotros are outside of the shoe. All regular forms are outside the shoe.

👣 👣 **GO VERBS-Verbs that have a go ending in the yo form**

**The Spanish "yo-go" verbs are as follows:**

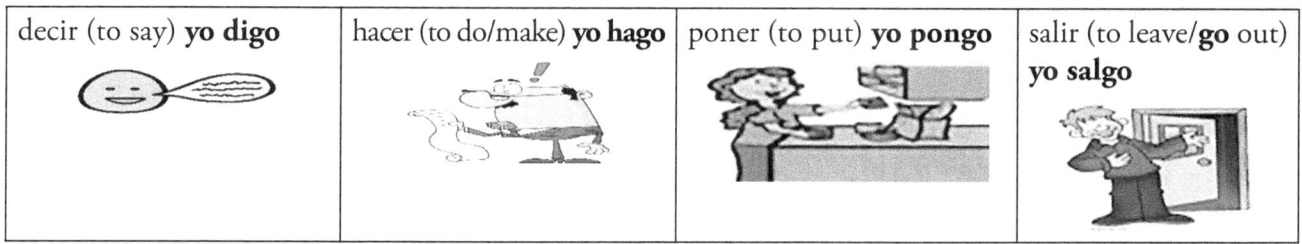

| decir (to say) **yo digo** | hacer (to do/make) **yo hago** | poner (to put) **yo pongo** | salir (to leave/**go** out) **yo salgo** |
|---|---|---|---|

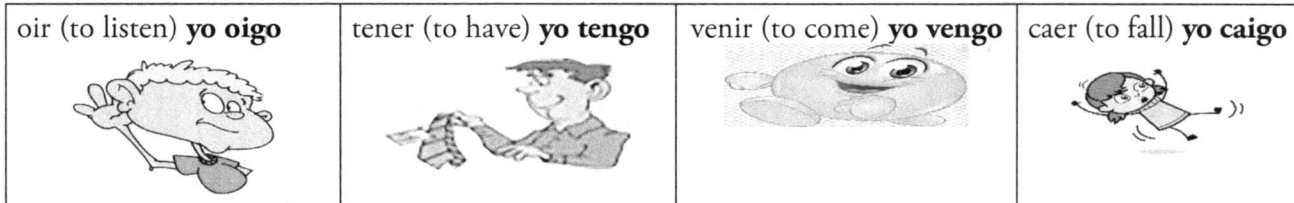

| oir (to listen) **yo oigo** | tener (to have) **yo tengo** | venir (to come) **yo vengo** | caer (to fall) **yo caigo** |

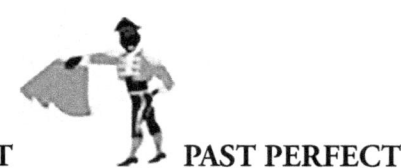

# PRESENT PERFECT    PAST PERFECT

**HABER-auxiliary verb**

| Yo | he | había |
|---|---|---|
| Tú | has | habías |
| Él, ella, Usted | ha | había |
| Nosotros | hemos | habíamos |
| Vosotros | habéis | habíais |
| Ellos, Ellas, Ustedes | han | habían |

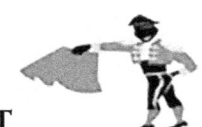

# PRESENT PERFECT

USE HABER + PAST PARTICIPLE (-ado for –ar verbs & -ido for -ir & -er verbs) Example: Juan ha comido. Juan has eaten. ✈ ☉ ☏ Yo he llamado a Juan. I have called Juan. ☎ Tú has vivido en México. You have lived in Mexico 🏠 🏠

# PAST PERFECT

USE HABER + PAST PARTICIPLE (-ado for –ar verbs & -ido for -ir & -er verbs)

Example: Juan había comido. Juan had eaten. ✈ ☉ ☏ Yo había llamado a Juan. I called Juan. ☎ Tú habías vivido en México. You had lived in Mexico 🏠 🏠

## PAST TENSE- PRETERIT & IMPERFECT

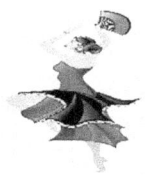

## PRETERIT

| Subject Pronoun | Habl-ar | Com-er | Viv-ir |
|---|---|---|---|
| Yo | Habl-é | Com-í | Viv-í |
| Tú | Habl-aste | Com-iste | Viv-iste |
| Él, ella, Usted | Habl-ó | Com-ió | Viv-ió |
| Nosotros | Habl-amos | Com-imos | Viv-imos |
| Vosotros | Habl-asteis | Com-isteis | Viv-isteis |
| Ellos, ellas, Ustedes | Habl-aron | Com-ieron | Viv-ieron |

OJO *take note* The preterit tense has two sets of endings: one for –ar verbs and the same for –er & -ir verbs for regular verbs. The nosotros for –ar is the same in the present tense and the preterit tense. Context determines which tense it is referring to. Ex-Hablamos con Juan todos los días- We speak with Juan every day. Ayer hablamos con Juan. We spoke with Juan yesterday.

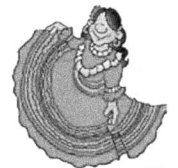

## PRETERIT IRREGULARS

|  | yo | tú | Él, ella, Usted | Nosotros, nosotras | Ellos, ellas, Ustedes |
|---|---|---|---|---|---|
| IR & SER | fui | Fuiste | fue | fuimos | fueron |
| DAR | di | diste | dio | dimos | dieron |
| VER | vi | viste | Vio | vimos | vieron |

OJO *take note* Ir and ser have the same preterit conjugation. Context determines which is being used. Ex-Juan fue al cine. Juan went to the movies. Juan fue simpático. Juan was nice.

## U-STEM PRETERIT IRREGULARS ❀

| ESTAR (u-stem) | estuve | estuviste | estuvo | estuvimos | estuvieron |
|---|---|---|---|---|---|
| TENER (u-stem) | tuve | tuviste | tuvo | tuvimos | tuvieron |
| ANDAR (u-stem) | anduve | anduviste | anduvo | anduvimos | anduvieron |
| PONER-(u-stem) | puse | pusiste | puso | pusimos | pusieron |
| SABER (u-stem) | supe | supiste | supo | supimos | supieron |
| PODER (u-stem) | pude | pudiste | pudo | pudimos | pudieron |

## I-STEM PRETERIT IRREGULARS ❀

| HACER (I-stem) | Hice | hiciste | hizo | hicimos | hicieron |
|---|---|---|---|---|---|
| QUERER (I-stem) | quise | quisiste | quiso | quisimos | quisieron |
| VENIR (I-stem) | vine | viniste | vino | vinimos | vinieron |

## J-STEM PRETERIT IRREGULARS ❀

| DECIR | dije | dijiste | dijo | dijimos | dijeron |
|---|---|---|---|---|---|
| TRAER | traje | trajiste | trajo | trajimos | trajeron |
| CONDUCIR | conduje | condujiste | condujo | condujimos | condujeron |

OJO *take note* The preterit has various irregular verbs. Among them are the : u-stem, i-stem and j-stem. The verbs endings for the i, j and u stem verbs are: -e. -iste, -o, -imos, -isteis and-ieron. There are no accents on any of the preterit -i,-j or –u stems. The –j stems 3rd person plural form is –eron. The 3rd person singular for hacer is hizo.

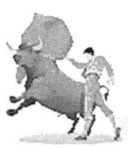

## IMPERFECT

| Subject Pronoun | Habl-ar | Com-er | Viv-ir |
|---|---|---|---|
| Yo | Habl-aba | Com-ía | Viv-ía |
| Tú | Habl-abas | Com-ías | Viv-ías |
| Él, ella, Usted | Habl-aba | Com-ía | Viv-ía |
| Nosotros | Habl-ábamos | Com-íamos | Viv-íamos |
| Vosotros | Habl-abais | Com-iais | Viv-iais |
| Ellos, ellas, Ustedes | Habl-aban | Com-ían | Viv-ían |

OJO take note The first & third person conjugations are the same in the imperfect. If the subject or subject pronoun is not listed, context will help you determine subject.

## IRREGULAR IMPERFECT

| Subject Pronoun | Ir | Ser | ver |
|---|---|---|---|
| Yo | iba | era | Veía |
| Tú | ibas | eras | Veías |
| Él, ella, Usted | iba | era | Veía |
| Nosotros | íbamos | eramos | Veíamos |
| Vosotros | ibáis | erais | Veiais |
| Ellos, ellas, Ustedes | iban | eran | Veían |

OJO take note The imperfect has only 3 irregulars: ir, ser and ver.

# PRETERIT VS IMPERFECT USES 🌷

| PRETERIT 🌸 past completed action with a clear beginning & a clear end.<br><br>Ex Yesterday I studied. Ayer estudié. | IMPERFECT 🌸 past repeated action, background action, time, age, whenever you would say 'was' or 'used to' in English<br><br>Ex Cuando era niño, estudiaba todos los días. When I was a kid, I used to study every day. |
| --- | --- |

ACRONYM FOR CHOOSING BETWEEN PRETERIT VS IMPERFECT

**SIMBA CHEATED**

PRETERIT- **SIMBA** (**S**ingle Action, **I**nterruption, **M**ain Event, **B**eginning Action, **A**rrivals/ Departures)

IMPERFECT- **CHEATED** (**C**haracteristics, **H**ealth, **E**motion, **A**ge, **T**ime, **E**ndless activities, **D**ate)

**FORMAL COMMANDS** (Formal command have only USTED & USTEDES forms)

OJO *take note* Go to the 'yo' form of a verb, drop the —o and add the opposite vowel (-e for —ar verbs & -a for —er and —ir verbs)

| SUBJECT | comprar | vender | escribir |
| --- | --- | --- | --- |
| USTED | compr-e | venda | escriba |
| USTEDES | compr-en | vendan | escriban |

OJO *take note* **There are 6 irregular Ud/Uds commands:** dar - to give: dé, den.

- estar - to be. esté, estén
- haber - to have (auxiliary verb) haya, hayan
- ir - to go. vaya, vayan
- saber - to know. sepa, sepa.
- ser - to be. sea, sean

# THE PRESENT SUBJUNCTIVE

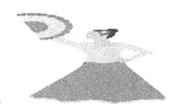

**OJO** To form the present subjunctive: go to the 'yo' form of a verb, drop the –o and add the opposite vowel (-e for –ar verbs & -a for –er and –ir verbs).

| Subject Pronoun | Habl-ar | Com-er | Viv-ir |
|---|---|---|---|
| Yo | Habl-e | Com-a | Viv-a |
| Tú | Habl-es | Com-as | Viv-as |
| Él, ella, Usted | Habl-e | Com-a | Viv-a |
| Nosotros | Habl-emos | Com-amos | Viv-amos |
| Vosotros | Habl-eis | Com-ais | Viv-ais |
| Ellos, ellas, Ustedes | Habl-en | Com-an | Viv-an |

**OJO** The present subjunctive is used when there are 2 separate clauses in a sentence and used when there is **wish, emotion or doubt ACRONYM: WEDDING**.

example-
**WISH**: I want Juan to study . Quiero que Juan estudie.
**EMOTION**: I hope Juan studies. Espero que Juan estudie.
**DOUBT:** I doubt that Juan will study. Dudo que Juan estudie.

# WORKBOOK EXERCISES

## INSTRUCTIONS FOR MEDICATIONS. PICK THE CORRECT WORD FROM WORDBANK

Nombre y dirección de la farmacia, medicamento, potencia y presentación, la fecha de expiración, cantidad de rellenos, el día que llega la receta, el fabricante del medicamento, instrucciones al paciente, el número de la receta, el nombre del doctor quien hace la receta, el nombre del paciente, cantidad recetada,

Instructions for medication, Instrucciones para medicamentos

Prescription Label,

3. Name & address of the pharmacy,

2. The name of the prescribing doctor,

1. Date of medication,

4. Number of the prescription,

5. Patient's name,

6. Medication/strength of the medicine/form of medication,

7. Prescribed quantity,

8. Number of refills,

**J** Jerry's Pharmacy
135 West 81st Street
New York, New York 21007

TELEPHONE NUMBER,
NÚMERO DE TELÉFONO: (555)555-5555

DR K. Vin Nortans

NO 0060023-08291
ANNA SIMMONS

DATE, FECHA: 05/05/22

123 Indiana Ave. New York, NY 11111
TAKE ONE CAPSULE BY
MOUTH TWO TIMES A DAY,
TOME UNA CÁPSULA POR BOCA 2 VECES
CADA DÍA

Take on an empty stomach, 1 hour before or 2-3 hours after eating.Tómese con el estómago vacío,1 hora antes o 2-3 horas después de comer.

CURALLACILLIN 500MG
CAPSULES

QTY 20    MFG XYZ
NO REFILLS, NO SE PERMITEN RELLENOS
You must see a doctor for refill. Usted debe ver
a un médico antes de que esta receta pueda ser rellenada.
USE BEFORE, USE ANTES DE:05/05/23
05/05/23

9. Drug manufacturer,

10. Instructions to the patient,

11. Expiration date,

**Choose the correct Spanish translation using the below wordbank.**

**MEDICATIONS MEDICAMENTOS. Please pick the correct word from the wordbank:**

El inhalador, las gotas para los ojos, el diurético, la cortisona, los analgésicos, la vitamina,el antigripal, los antiácidos, el laxante, el esteroide, la pomada, el supositorio, el jarabe para la tos, los antibióticos, el sedante, el estrógeno, los antisépticos, la penicilina, el descongestionante, el antidepresivo, los medicamentos de venta libre, los anithistamínicos, los tranquilizantes/los calmantes, la aspirina, el expectorante, la insulina

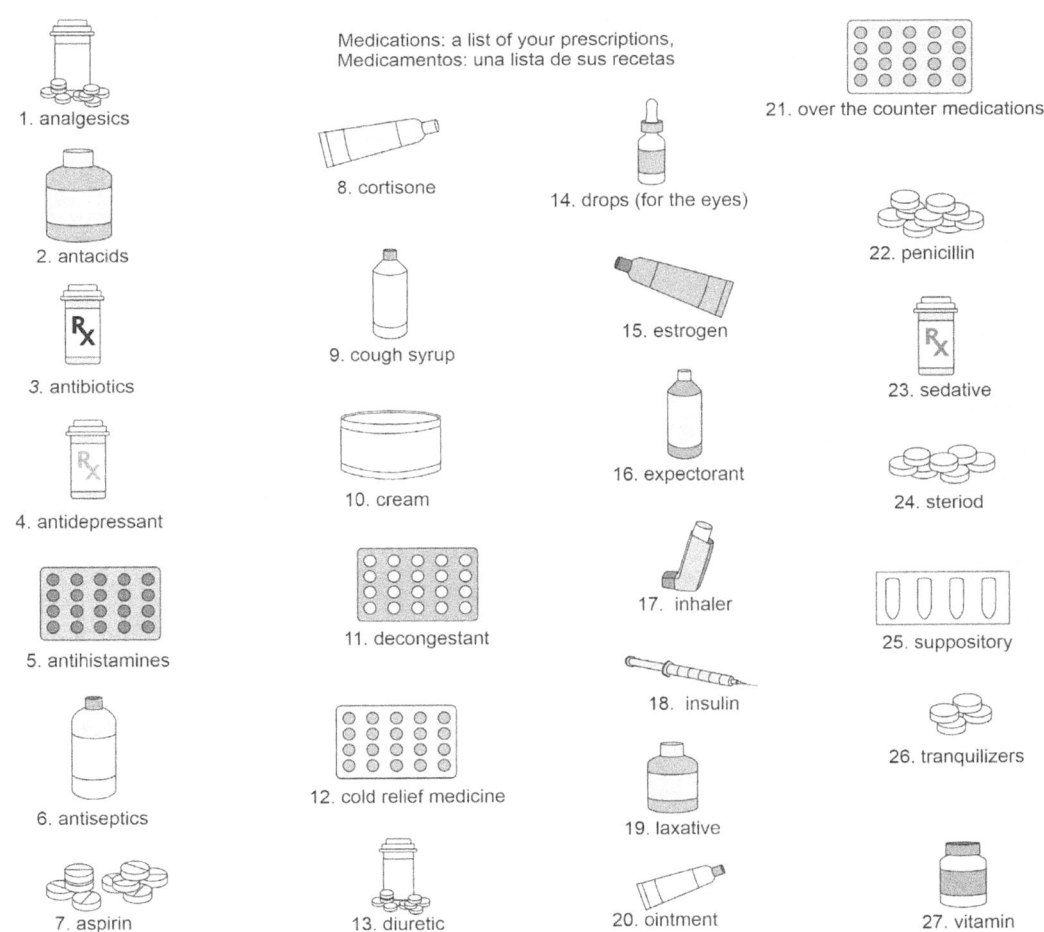

Medications: a list of your prescriptions,
Medicamentos: una lista de sus recetas

1. analgesics

2. antacids

3. antibiotics

4. antidepressant

5. antihistamines

6. antiseptics

7. aspirin

8. cortisone

9. cough syrup

10. cream

11. decongestant

12. cold relief medicine

13. diuretic

14. drops (for the eyes)

15. estrogen

16. expectorant

17. inhaler

18. insulin

19. laxative

20. ointment

21. over the counter medications

22. penicillin

23. sedative

24. steriod

25. suppository

26. tranquilizers

27. vitamin

**Choose the correct Spanish translation using the below word bank.**

<u>**UNITS OF MEASURE:**</u>

la taza dosificadora, la cuchara dosificadora, la jeringa, las tabletas, la cápsula, el vertidor de medicina, las pastillas, las bocanadas, la jeringa oral

<u>**STORAGE FOR MEDICATIONS:**</u>

Lejos de la calefacción, en un lugar seco, guera de la luz del sol, en el refrigerador, al tempo, lejos del alcance de los niños

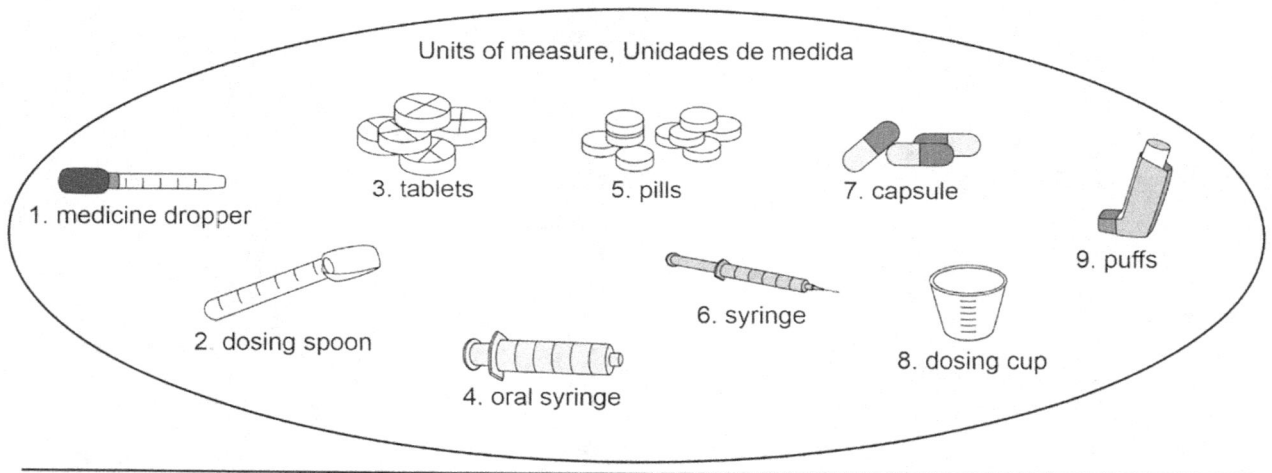

Units of measure, Unidades de medida

1. medicine dropper
2. dosing spoon
3. tablets
4. oral syringe
5. pills
6. syringe
7. capsule
8. dosing cup
9. puffs

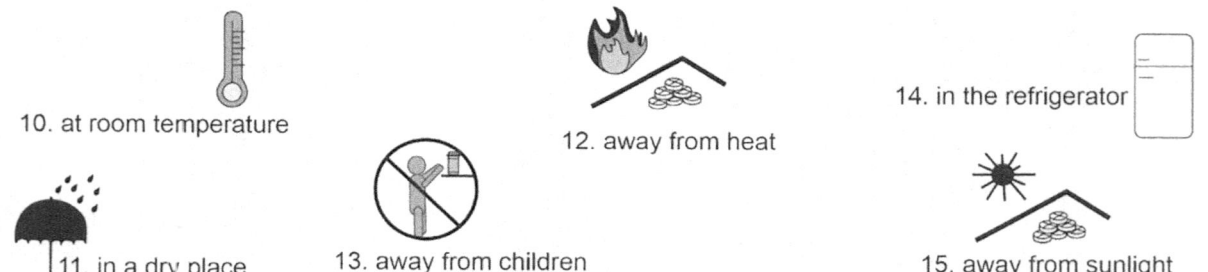

Medicine storage, Almacenamiento de medicamentos

10. at room temperature
11. in a dry place
12. away from heat
13. away from children
14. in the refrigerator
15. away from sunlight

**Choose the correct Spanish translation using the below wordbank.**

**Pharmacy/Rx Vocabulary**

La farmacia por correo, la versión genérica, las recetas de venta libre, la farmacia, los medicamentos con receta, los medicamentos, la receta, el/la farmaceútico/a

**Methods of Ingestion**

Bomba/bombilla, masticar, uso oral, el inyectable, poner gotas, inhaladores nasales, inhalar, inhaladores orales, uso nasal, el inhalador, tragar

**Frequency**

__veces al día, por la mañana, por la tarde, por la noche, cada _____ horas, antes de comer/con cada comida/después de comer, un día sí, un día no, cada tercer día

**How to Take Medication**

Con mucho agua, no tome con alcohol, en ayunas/túmeselo con el estómago vacío, no tome leche o productos lácteos meintras esté tomando esta medicina, no lo mastique

**Warnings**

Masticar antes de tragar

Manténgase refrigerado

Agítese bien antes de usalro

Necesita tomar toda la medicina

Mantenga los medicamentos fuera del alcance de los niños

Evite exponerse al sol meintras esté tomando la medicina

**Side effects**

Diarrea, dolor estomacal, mareos, somnolencia, este medicamento puede afectar la capacidad para conducir, boca seca

**Refills/ Expiration**

Esta receta no pude rellenarse, medicamentos caducos, no use después de, fecha de caducidad/fecha de vencimiento, deséchese después de.., esta receta puede__rellenados

# Instructions for medication, Instrucciones para medicamentos

## Pharmacy/Rx vocabulary
1. generic version,
2. medications,
3. on-line pharmacy,
4. over-the-counter medications,
5. pharmacist,
6. pharmacy,
7. prescription,
8. prescription drugs,

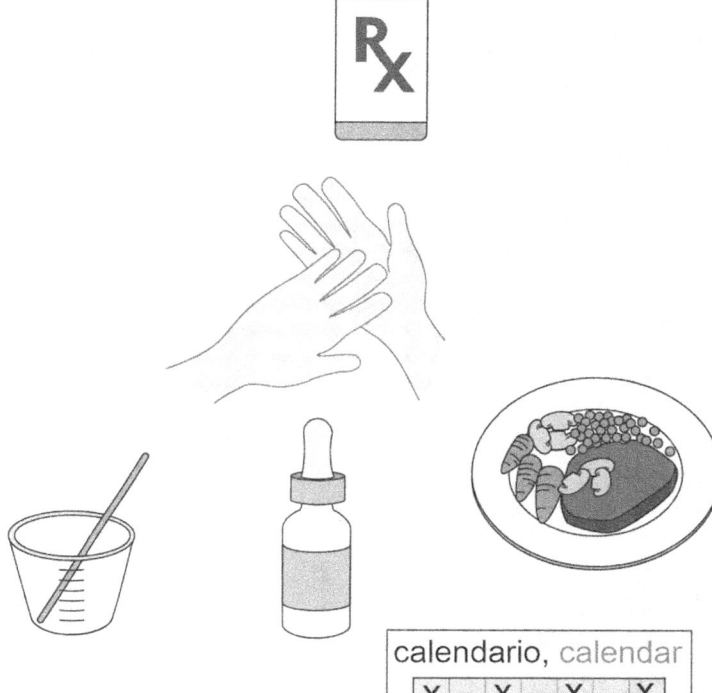

## Method of ingestion,
9. To swallow,
10. To chew,
11. To put drops in eyes,
12. To inhale,
13. Inhaler,
14. Injectable,
15. Nasal use,
16. Nasal inhalers,
17. Oral inhalers,
18. Oral use,
19. Pump,

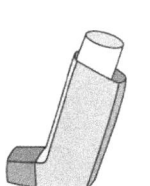

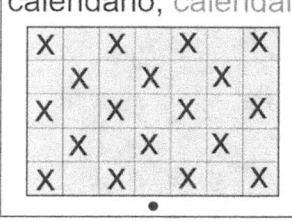

## Frequency,
20. Take this medicine…,
21. ____times a day,
22. Every day…every other day…..,
23 very___hours,
24. in the morning/evening,
25. Before eating /with each meal/after eating…, antes de comer/con cada comida/después de comer24.

## How to Take Medication,
26. On an empty stomach,
27. With plenty of water,
28. Don't chew; swallow,
29. Don't take with alcohol.
30. Don't drink milk or dairy products while taking this medication.

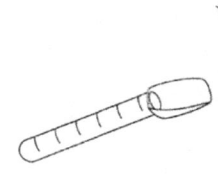

## Warnings,
31. Avoid staying in the sun while taking this medicine.
32. Chew pills before swallowing.
33. Keep in a cool place.
34. Keep out of reach of children.
35. Keep refrigerated.
36. Shake well before using.
37. You need to take all of the medicine.

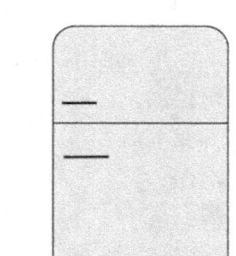

## Side effects,
38. This medicine can cause...,
39. diarrhea,
40. dizziness,
41. drowsiness,
42. dry mouth,
43. stomach pain,
44. This medicine can impair driving,

## Refills/Expiration,
45. Expired medication,
46. Expiration date,
47. This medicine does not have refills.
48. Throw out after _____,
49. There can be _____ refills.
50. Don't use after _____,

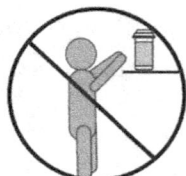

# WORDBANK. CHOOSE THE CORRECT SPANISH TRANSLATION

Este RX puede rellenarse como sea necesario, puede causar somnolencia, no tome con jugo; tome con agua o leche; favor de no tirar medicamentos no utilizados en el drenaje o el lavabo, Tómese con bastante agua, uso externo, no tome por la boca, no use después de FECHA:no tome por la boca, para uso externo,Importante:Termine todo este medicamento a menos que su médico le indique lo contrario, este RX sólo se puede rellenar por autoridad de su médico por un servicio más rápido, llámenos para rellenar durante sus horas de oficina, no tome bebidas alcohólicas mientras se usa,agítese bien y manténgase en el refrigerador

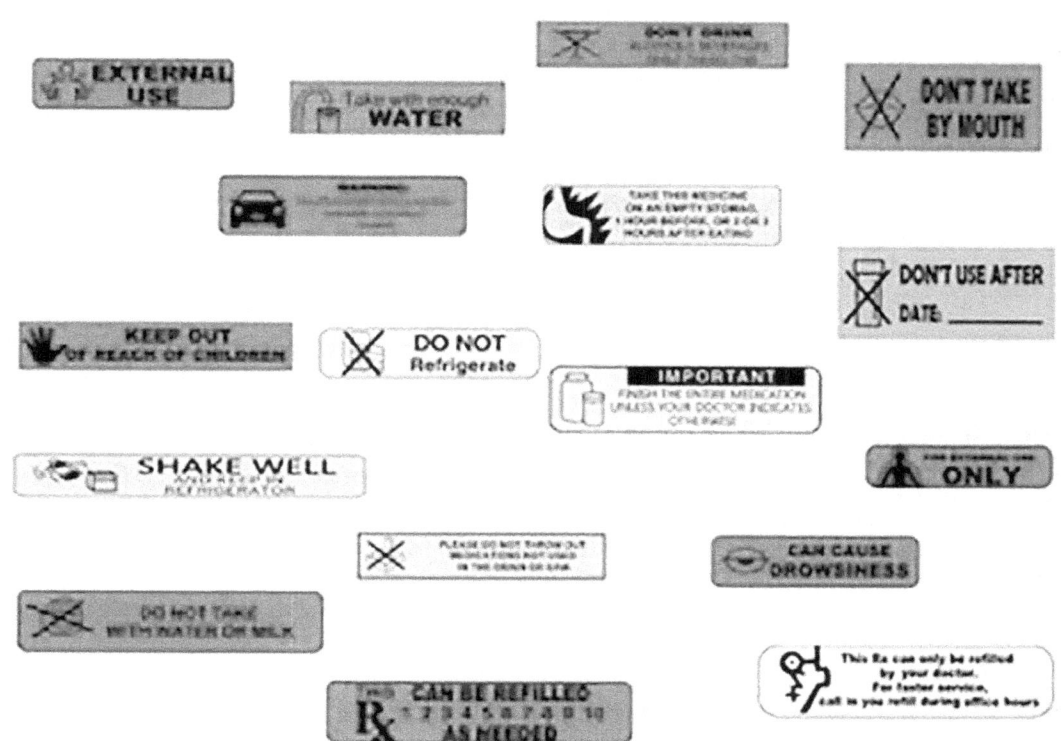

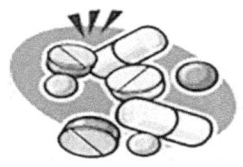 **MEDICATIONS** PICK THE CORRECT WORD FROM WORDBANK.

tranquilizante, supositorio, unguento, penicilina, aspirina, antisépticos, jarabe para la tos, estrógeno, analgésicos, diurético, gotas para los ojos, antigripal

a) suppository _____

b) penicillin_____

c)diuretic_____

d)antiseptics_____

e) analgesics_____

f) estrogen_____

g) cold relief medicine_____

h) eye drops _____

i) aspirin_____

j) ointment_____

k) tranquilizers_____

l) cough syrup_____

**The First Aid Kit. El Botiquín de primeros auxilios.**

guantes (desechables o descartables), una mascarilla de reanimación cardiopulmonar, antiinflamatorios, antidiarréicos, jabón desinfectante, crema para picaduras, almohadillas de alcohol, lista de teléfonos de emergencia, aspirina, crema de hidrocortisona, peróxido de hidrógeno, crema para quemaduras, jarabe, yodo, curitas, gasa estéril, bajalenguas, manual de primeros auxilios, esparadrapo, mascarillas desechables o descartables, gotas de colirio-monodósis, jeringas desechables o descartables, venda de gasa, antisépticos, tijeras, antiácidos, pinzas, termómetro, una linterna con baterías de repuesto, algodón, unguento antibiótico , crema para lesiones

# First aid kit, Botiquín de primeros auxilios

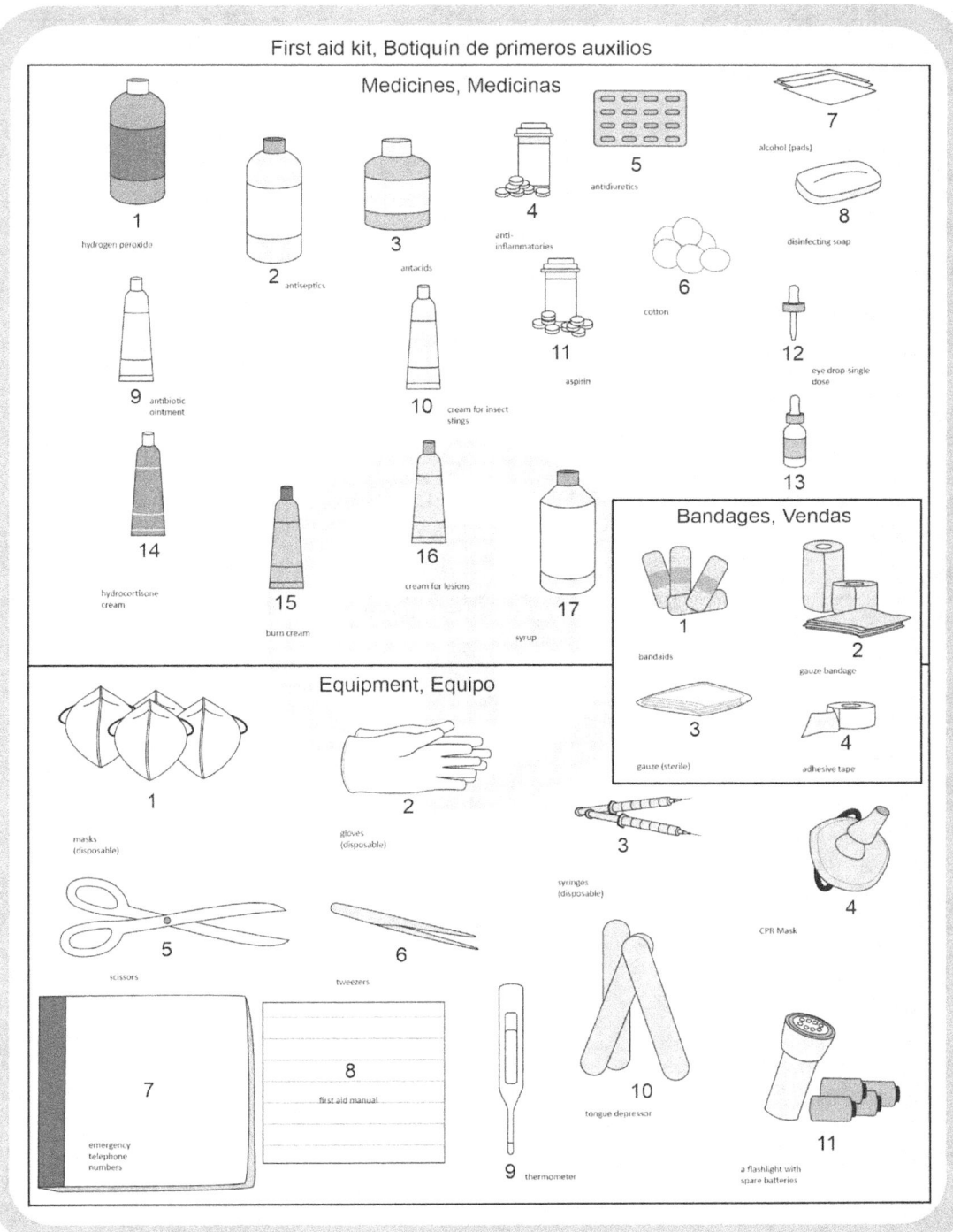

## Medicines, Medicinas

1. hydrogen peroxide
2. antiseptics
3. antacids
4. anti-inflammatories
5. antidiuretics
6. cotton
7. alcohol (pads)
8. disinfecting soap
9. antibiotic ointment
10. cream for insect stings
11. aspirin
12. eye drop-single dose
13.
14. hydrocortisone cream
15. burn cream
16. cream for lesions
17. syrup

## Bandages, Vendas

1. bandaids
2. gauze bandage
3. gauze (sterile)
4. adhesive tape

## Equipment, Equipo

1. masks (disposable)
2. gloves (disposable)
3. syringes (disposable)
4. CPR Mask
5. scissors
6. tweezers
7. emergency telephone numbers
8. first aid manual
9. thermometer
10. tongue depressor
11. a flashlight with spare batteries

---

Instructions for medication, Instrucciones para medicamentos

Prescription Label, La etiqueta

1. Date of medication, el día que llega la receta
2. The name of the prescribing doctor, el nombre del doctor quien hace la receta
3. Name & address of the pharmacy, nombre y dirección de la farmacia
4. Number of the prescription, el número de la receta
5. Patient's name, el nombre del paciente
6. Medication/strength of the medicine/form of medication, medicamento, potencia y presentación
7. Prescribed quantity, cantidad recetada
8. Number of refills, cantidad de rellenos
9. Drug manufacturer, el fabricante del medicamento
10. Instructions to the patient, instrucciones al paciente
11. Expiration date, la fecha de expiración

---

Medications: a list of your prescriptions, Medicamentos: una lista de sus recetas

1. analgesics, los analgésicos
2. antacids, los antiácidos
3. antibiotics, los antibióticos
4. antidepressant, el antidepresivo
5. antihistamines, los antihistamínicos
6. antiseptics, los antisépticos
7. aspirin, la aspirina

8. cortisone, la cortisona
9. cough syrup, el jarabe para la tos
10. cream, la pomada
11. decongestant, el descongestionante
12. cold relief medicine, el antigripal
13. diuretic, el diurético

14. drops (for the eyes), las gotas (para los ojos)
15. estrogen, el estrógeno
16. expectorant, el expectorante
17. inhaler, el inhalador
18. insulin, la insulina
19. laxative, el laxante
20. ointment, el ungüento

21. over the counter medications, los medicamentos de venta libre
22. penicillin, la penicilina
23. sedative, el sedante
24. steriod, el esteroide
25. suppository, el supositorio
26. tranquilizers, los tranquilizantes, los calmantes
27. vitamin, la vitamina

Units of measure, Unidades de medida

1. medicine dropper, vertidor de medicina
2. dosing spoon, cuchara dosificadora
3. tablets, las tabletas
4. oral syringe, la jeringa oral
5. pills, las pastillas
6. syringe, la jeringa
7. capsule, la cápsula
8. dosing cup, la taza dosificadora
9. puffs, las bocanadas

Medicine storage, Almacenamiento de medicamentos

10. at room temperature,  al tiempo
11. in a dry place, en un lugar seco
12. away from heat, en un lugar seco
13. away from children, lejos del alcance de los niños
14. in the refrigerator, en el refrigerador
15. away from sunlight, fuera de la luz del sol

Instructions for medication, Instrucciones para medicamentos

Pharmacy/Rx vocabulary
1. generic version,
2. medications,
3. on-line pharmacy,
4. over-the-counter medications,
5. pharmacist,
6. pharmacy,
7. prescription,
8. prescription drugs,

Method of ingestion,
9. To swallow,
10. To chew,
11. To put drops in eyes,
12. To inhale,
13. Inhaler,
14. Injectable,
15. Nasal use,
16. Nasal inhalers,
17. Oral inhalers,
18. Oral use,
19. Pump,

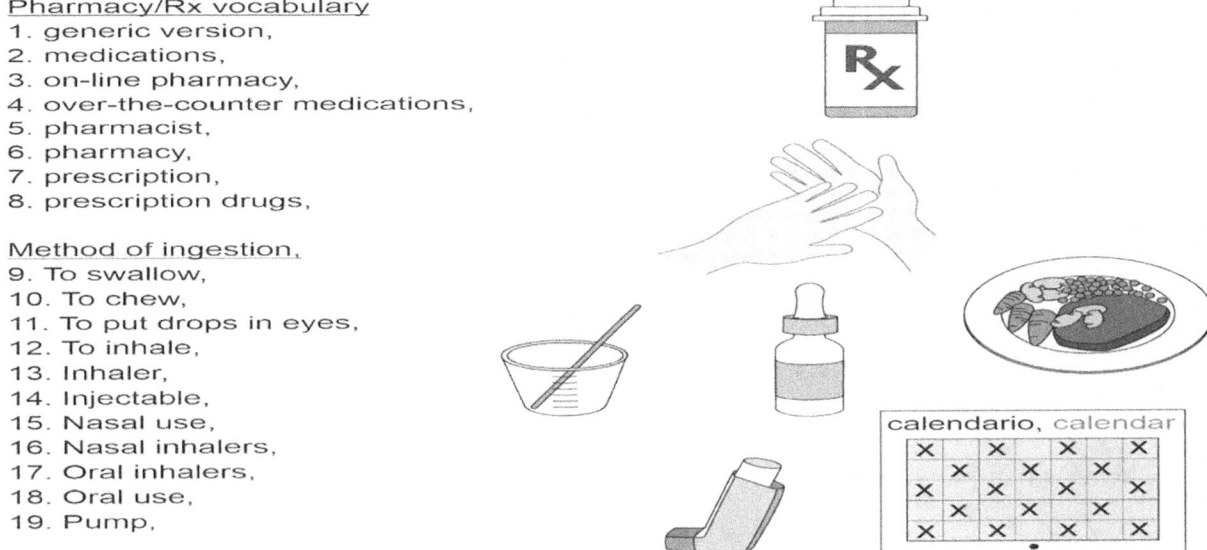

Frequency,
20. Take this medicine…,
21. _____times a day,
22. Every day…every other day…..,
23 very____hours,
24. in the morning/evening,
25. Before eating /with each meal/after eating…, antes de comer/con cada comida/después de comer

How to take medications Instrucciones para tomar la medicación

26. on an empty stomach

27. with plenty of water

28. don't chew / swallow

29. don't take with alcohol

30. don't drink milk or dairy products while taking this medication

## Warnings advertencias

31. Avoid staying in the sun while taking this medicine.

32. Chew pills before swallowing.

33. Keep in a cool place.

34. Keep out of reach of children.

35. Keep refrigerated.

36. Shake well before using.

37. You need to take all of the medicine.

## Side effects

38. This medicine can cause..

39. diarrhea

40. diziness

41. drowsiness

42. dry mouth

43. stomach pain

44. This medicine can impair driving.

## Refills/expiration Rellenos / Fecha de caducidad

45. expired medication

46. Expired date

47. This medicine does not have refills.

48. Throw out after...

49. There can be _____ refills.

50. Do not use after_____

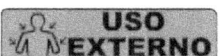

**USO EXTERNO**

External use

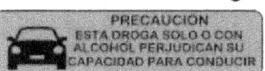

TÓMESE CON BASTANTE **AGUA**

Take with enough water

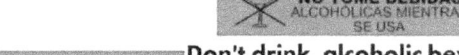

**NO TOME BEBIDAS**
ALCOHÓLICAS MIENTRAS SE USA

Don't drink alcoholic beverages while taking this

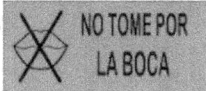

NO TOME POR LA BOCA

Don't take by mouth

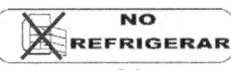

PRECAUCIÓN
ESTA DROGA SOLO O CON ALCOHOL PERJUDICAN SU CAPACIDAD PARA CONDUCIR

**Warning:**
This drug alone or with alcohol can harm your hability to drive

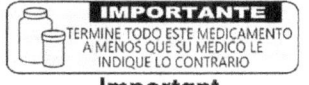

TOME ESTA MEDICINA CON EL ESTÓMAGO VACIO 1 HORA ANTES O 2 Ó 3 HORAS DESPUES DE COMER

Take this medicine on an empty stomach, 1 hour before, or 2 or 3, hours after eating

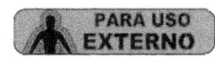

NO USE DESPUES DE FECHA: _____

Don't use after
Date: _____

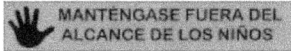

MANTÉNGASE FUERA DEL ALCANCE DE LOS NIÑOS

Keep out of reach of children

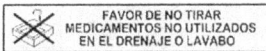

**NO REFRIGERAR**

Do not refrigerate

**IMPORTANTE**
TERMINE TODO ESTE MEDICAMENTO A MENOS QUE SU MEDICO LE INDIQUE LO CONTRARIO

Important
Finish the entire medication unless your doctor indicates otherwise

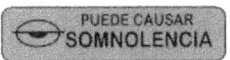

PARA USO **EXTERNO**

For external use

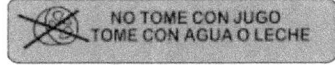

**AGÍTESE BIEN**
Y MANTÉNGASE EN REFRIGERADOR

Shake well and keep in refrigerator

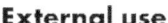

FAVOR DE NO TIRAR MEDICAMENTOS NO UTILIZADOS EN EL DRENAJE O LAVABO

Please do not throw out medications not used in the drain or sink

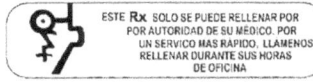

PUEDE CAUSAR **SOMNOLENCIA**

Can cause drowsiness

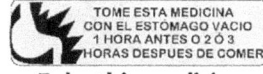

NO TOME CON JUGO TOME CON AGUA O LECHE

Do not take with water or milk

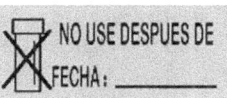

ESTE **Rx** PUEDE RELLENARSE 1 2 3 4 5 6 7 8 9 10 COMO SEA NECESARIO

Can be refilled as needed

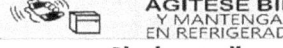

ESTE **Rx** SOLO SE PUEDE RELLENAR POR POR AUTORIDAD DE SU MÉDICO. POR UN SERVICIO MAS RAPIDO, LLAMENOS RELLENAR DURANTE SUS HORAS DE OFICINA

This RX can only be refilled by your doctor for faster service, call in your refill during office hours

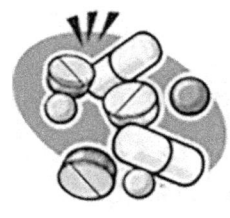

**MEDICATIONS** PICK THE CORRECT WORD FROM WORDBANK.

a) supositorio

b) penicilina

c) diurético

d) antisépticos

e) analgésicos

f) estrógeno

g) el antigripal

h) gotas para los ojos

i) aspirina

J) unguento

k) tranquilizantes

l) jarabe para la tos

First aid kit, Botiquín de primeros auxilios

## Medicines, Medicinas

1. hydrogen peroxide, peróxido de hidrógeno
2. antiseptics, antisépticos
3. antacids, antiácidos
4. anti-inflammatories, antiinflamatorios
5. antidiuretics, antidiarréicos
6. cotton, algodón
7. alcohol (pads), alcohol (almohadillas de alcohol)
8. disinfecting soap, jabón desinfecante
9. antibiotic ointment, unguento antibiótico
10. cream for instinct stings, crema para picaduras
11. aspirin, aspirina
12. eye drops-single dose, gotas de colirio-monodósis
13. iodine, yodo
14. hydrocortizone cream, crema de hidrocortisona
15. burn cream, crema para quemaduras
16. cream for lesions, crema para lesiones
17. syrup, járabe

## Equipment, Equipo

1. masks (disposable), mascarillas desechables o descartables
2. gloves (disposable), guantes (desechables or descartables)
3. syringes (disposable), jeringes (desechables or descartables)
4. a cpr mask, una mascarilla de reanimación cardiopulmonar
5. scissors, tijeras
6. tweezers, pinzas
7. first aid manual, manual de primeros auxilios
8. emergency phone numbers, lista de teléfonos de emergencia
9. thermometer, termómetro
10. tongue depressor, bajalenguas
11. a flashlight with spare batteries, una linterna con baterías de repuesto

## Bandages, Vendas

1. bandaids, curitas
2. gauze bandage, venda de gasa
3. gauze (sterile), gasa estéril,
4. adhesive tape, esparadrapo,